TOPICS IN SPINAL ANAESTHESIA

Edited by **Victor M. Whizar-Lugo**

Topics in Spinal Anaesthesia
http://dx.doi.org/10.5772/57013
Edited by Victor M. Whizar-Lugo

Contributors

Alparslan Apan, R. Hakan Erbay, Nimet Senoglu, Habip Atalay, Víctor Whizar-Lugo, Juan C. Flores-Carrillo, Susana Preciado-Ramírez, Víctor Silva, Jaime Campos-León, Nicola Nicassio, Irfan Malik, Hala Mostafa Goma, Amr Aboela, Beyazit Zencirci, W. Scott Jellish, Steven Edelstein

Published by InTech

Janeza Trdine 9, 51000 Rijeka, Croatia

Publishing Process Manager Iva Lipovic

Technical Editor InTech DTP team

Cover InTech Design team

First published August, 2014

Printed in Croatia

Additional hard copies can be obtained from orders@intechopen.com

Topics in Spinal Anaesthesia, Edited by Victor M. Whizar-Lugo

p. cm.

ISBN 978-953-51-1720-9

For EU product safety concerns:
IN TECH d.o.o., Prolaz Marije Krucifikse Kozulić 3, 51000 Rijeka, Croatia,
info@intechopen.com or visit our website at intechopen.com.

Meet the editor

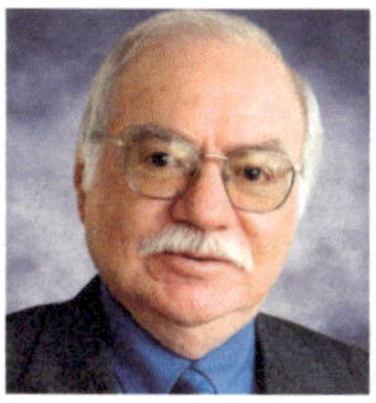

Victor M. Whizar-Lugo graduated from Universidad Nacional Autónoma de México, completed his residency in Internal Medicine at Hospital General de México, Anaesthesiology and Critical Care Medicine at Instituto Nacional de la Nutrición in México City, and Fellowship at the Anesthesia Department, Pain Clinic at University of California, Los Angeles, USA. Currently he works at the ICU of Hospital General de Tijuana, ISESALUD. He belongs to the Institutos Nacionales de Salud as associated researcher. He has more than 130 publications on anesthesia, pain, internal medicine and critical care journals/books. He has been a member of various editorial committees in anesthesiology journals, and was chief editor of the journal Anestesia en México. Dr. Whizar-Lugo is the founding director and current president of Anestesiología y Medicina del Dolor, a free medical educative program on the internet.

Contents

Preface

Spinal anaesthesia was described by Professor August Karl Gustav Bier just over a century ago. Since then, this technique has evolved and holds a special place in the current practice of worldwide anaesthesiology. Novel local anaesthetics with long acting duration and lower toxic potential, introduction of improved spinal needles, as well as the increasing use of old and new adjuvant drugs that improve the quality and duration of spinal anaesthesia and effective postoperative analgesia. All of these factors are the most important reasons that favor the use of this technique. Furthermore, spinal anaesthesia is safe, inexpensive, and easy to perform.

The authors of this book discussed various current topics on subarachnoid anaesthesia that are especially interesting and controversial due to the latest developments on this subject. *Topics on Spinal Anaesthesia* is a book composed by eight chapters addressing orthopaedic mayor surgery, ambulatory and short stay plastic surgery, complications, and subarachnoid drugs to enhance the effect of spinal local anaesthetics, as well as to provide prolonged post-operative analgesia.

As the editor, I thank the authors for their chapters, Gerardo Estolano-Ojeda HB for his support reviewing each chapter, and special thank to my two co-editors Juan Carlos Flores-Carrillo MD and Susana Preciado-Ramirez MD, for being the most energetic collaborators of this book. And last but not least, I thank my patients and my beloved family.

Víctor M. Whizar-Lugo MD
Intensive Care Unit
Hospital General de Tijuana, ISESALUD
Tijuana BC, México

Chapter 1

Spinal Anaesthesia in Spinal Surgery

Nicola Nicassio and Irfan Malik

Additional information is available at the end of the chapter

http://dx.doi.org/10.5772/58749

1. Introduction

Surgery for lumbar disc prolapse is one of the most common spinal procedures. Lumbar microdiscectomy is usually performed under general anaesthesia despite recent publications showed that these procedures can be performed safely also under spinal anaesthesia. Indeed, some authors have previously highlighted the possibility of using spinal anaesthesia for decompressive laminectomy and microdiscectomy, so avoiding the risks related to the general anaesthesia and allowing to reduce the length of the inpatient stay and the overall costs. In this chapter we will also expose different surgical procedures performed with local and general anaesthesia as well and we will give the possibility to the reader to realize the mean important differences with the use of the spinal anaesthesia.

2. Body

Spinal surgery is one of the more highly widespread disciplines in the world and it involves many different procedures, ranging from the easiest to the most complex ones.

In 1934 Mixter and Barr were the first authors to treat a lumbar disc herniation surgically by performing an open laminectomy and discectomy. With the introduction of the microscope, Caspar and Yasargil refined the original laminectomy into an open microdiscectomy.

Currently lumbar laminectomy and microdiscectomy, performed as open procedures by a posterior approach, are the most widespread procedure for surgical decompression.

Despite results are essentially related to the right indication for surgery and not to the anaesthetic or surgical techniques chosen, some complications are more correlated to the surgical approach and to the anaesthesiologist methods used.

For this reason in the last decades the technologies and the spinal surgeon's efforts have been addressed toward the use of the most minimally invasive procedures that can preserve as much as possible the anatomy in order to reduce the short-term and the long-term (post-operative fibrosis) surgical complications.

This is particularly true for the easiest spinal procedures as discectomy and central canal and foraminal decompression and all the new technical procedures, which have been developed, have allowed reaching two different aims:

a. To preserve as much as possible the anatomy of the whole spine (paravertebral muscles and ligaments included). With this objective in mind, minimally invasive and percutaneous approaches have been developed in order to reduce the damage to the anatomical structures and at the same time the intraoperative bleeding, the post-operative pain (and consequently the need of post-operative analgesia and related side effects), the incidence of post-operative infections and, eventually, the long-term post-operative fibrosis.

b. To lower the use of general anaesthesia and consequently all the risks related to its use. Indeed, the increase of the average age of the population has created a new class of patients that are more at risks of systemic (cardiovascular and pulmonary) complications.

Thus, in the last years, research and technology have pointed towards these two objectives, sometimes aiming for one in particular and, more rarely, achieving both of them. Particularly in the latter case, the result allows to manage the entire situation in the best way with clear consequences on the post-operative recovery period, which is often so fast to allow discharging the patient the same day of the operation. Evident implications arise on the economic benefits, as well.

Despite a detailed description of every surgical procedure falls outside the purpose of this chapter, we consider it useful to touch on the procedures that, in particular in the last period, have started to spread among the spinal surgeons. This will allow a clear understanding of the advantages and drawbacks as well as indications and contraindications of each procedure and to compare each other and all against the use of regional anaesthesia in spinal surgery.

Among the procedures that aimed for the goals in point a), a particular mention has to be done to the spinal endoscopy.

Spinal endoscopy was born as acting as a counterpart to the open spinal surgery and, since its introduction, has been applied for disc prolapse and stenosis of the entire spine, from the cervical to the lumbar segment [1].

Spinal endoscopy uses the "keyhole" rule, which is a specific entrance point where it is possible to insert progressive dilator tubes in order to create a way in which, at the end, it is possible to insert the endoscope.

Then, the endoscope allows having a wide view of the field (generally a 25° optic is used) and, makes it possible to insert and to work with surgical instruments, generally the same ones used for the open procedures. On the cervical spine, currently the authors prefer to perform the endoscopic procedure with the patient under general anaesthesia and an anterior (like the

http://dx.doi.org/10.5772/58749

anterior approach for the ACDF), or a posterior approach is used. Compared with the anterior approach [2], the posterior one is preferred because it is considered safer and less laden with major complications as injuries of the nervous-vascular bundle (ICA, internal jugular vein and vagus nerve) or of the esophagus [2, 3].

In addition, the corridor created, despite narrow, allows the surgeon to reach the disc and to remove it in small fragments without making any dangerous compression on the spinal cord.

Endoscopic techniques for the lumbar spine have been developed following different schools of thought which distinguish each other mainly: 1) on the endoscope's entry point (midline, postero-lateral and far-lateral) and 2) on the preferred anaesthesiologist techniques (local anaesthesia+mild sedation or general anaesthesia).

Of course, the decision about these variables depends on the pathology to face with (disc prolapse or central canal stenosis), the exact level of the disease (L5-S1 is considered a level for which some approach are not suitable) and the positioning of the pathology (midline, paramedian, foraminal, far lateral). Moreover, it is fundamental the surgeon's experience (who generally tends to use always the same approach) as the patient's condition, his past medical history and his ability to cooperate with the surgeon during the awake procedures.

The patient is in a prone or a lateral decubitus and this essentially depends on the approach used (the prone position usually requires the patient under general anaesthesia).

The postero-lateral and the far-lateral approaches allow reaching the pathology (generally a disc prolapse) passing through the foramen (transforaminal approach), with the endoscope which is located in the caudal half of the foramen (triangle safe zone) and the nerve root laying in the rostral half (Fig.1 and Fig 3).

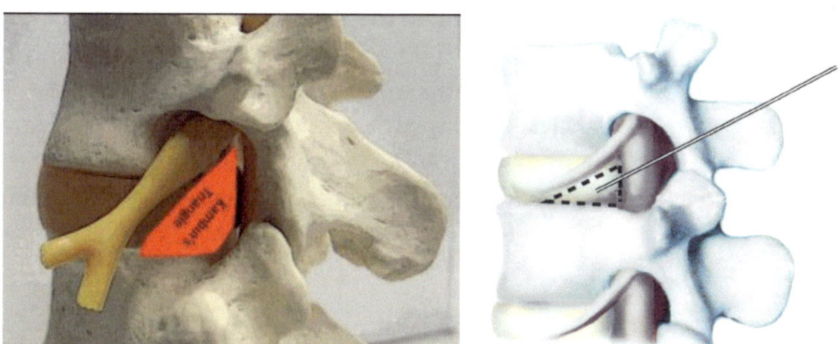

Figure 1. Triangle safe zone for the endoscopic transforaminal approach

The midline approach, on the contrary, is performed introducing the endoscope almost on the midline (roughly 2-3 mm laterally to avoid injury to the supraspinous ligament or to the interspinous ligament).

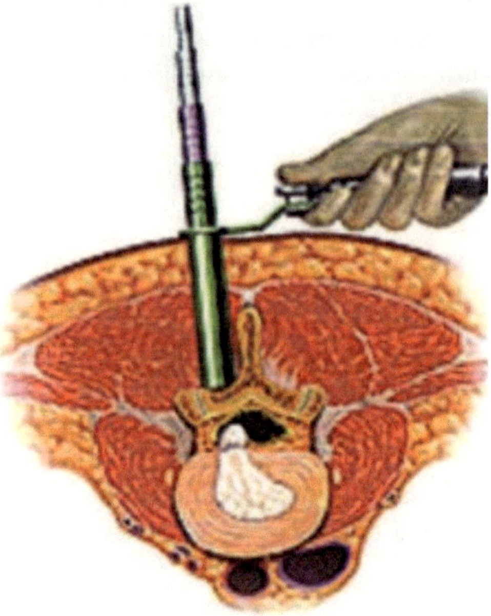

Figure 2. Midline endoscopic approach

With this approach, of course, it is necessary to remove some of the flavum ligament and part of the upper lamina and to dislodge medially the dural sac to reach the disc. The other approaches, on the contrary, allow reaching the disc without disrupting the flavum ligament and so reducing a lot the possibility of dura mater injury.

The transforaminal approach, generally with the patient on the lateral decubitus, can be performed under local anaesthesia and mild sedation or under general anaesthesia. The different choose is relevant in the positioning of the endoscope (this step of the procedure is done under fluoroscopic guide) and is dictated by some factors which are also related to the surgeon's personal experience and to the patient. The possibility to monitor the safe transit of the endoscope through the foramen by asking to the patient about the onset of any radicular pain is a tool that some surgeons are keen to use and for which, of course, the patient needs to be alert and completely collaborative (during this phase of the procedure the sedation needs to be stopped). This method can help to avoid damage to the nerve root during the position of the foramen [1, 5, 6].

Other surgeons prefer to ground only on the information given by the fluoroscopy and by a direct endoscopic vision of the nerve root and, for this reason, it is not necessary to work with an awake patient.

The midline approach is generally performed with the patient in the prone position and under general anaesthesia. The risk of a nerve root damage is quite small if compared with the transforaminal approach but the possibility of a dural tear and a consecutive dural fistula is more frequent.

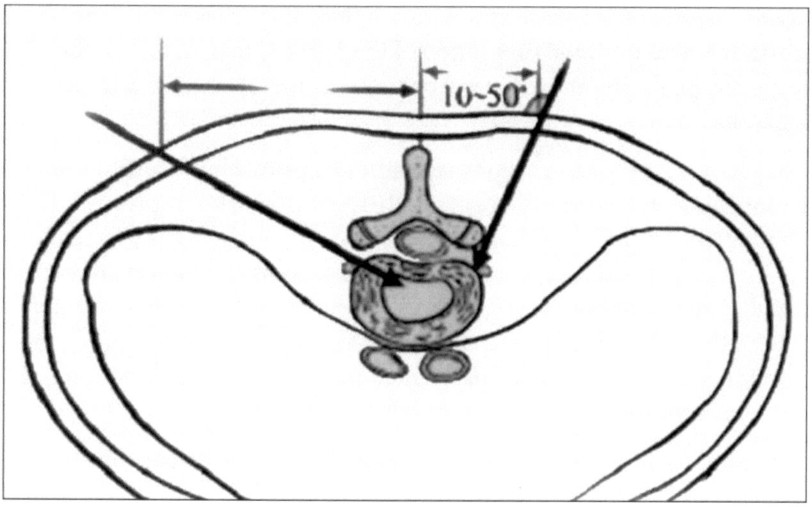

Figure 3. Different endoscope's direction in the transforaminal approach

The most suitable approach also depends on the axial position of the disc prolapse. Indeed, in case of a far lateral disc prolapse, a transforaminal approach is the most suitable to remove the compression while a foraminal disc herniation with a dislodgment of the nerve root caudally makes the transforaminal approach impossible to use or at least very dangerous.

About the sagittal position of the disc prolapsed, a migrated fragment behind the vertebral body is considered by some authors an absolute contraindication in performing endoscopic discectomy.

The surgeon's personal experience is another factor that should be considered, as some surgeons prefer to use always the same approach, not modifying it on the base of the level of the pathology or its axial position, while others prefer to change the approach according to the lumbar level interested in or the axial position of the compression. Thus, some surgeons face with the midline disc prolapse using a transforaminal approach while others prefer to use a midline approach.

The L5-S1 space is considered, by the majority of the authors a contraindication for the transforaminal approach because of the hindrance created by the iliac crest in conjunction with the inclination of this space. Despite these factors, some authors are keen to use the transforaminal approach and, relying on their great experience, in many cases are able to reach the L5-S1 space through this approach with the patient on the lateral decubitus and under local anaesthesia and mild sedation. Of course a high position of the iliac crest is an absolute contraindication to the transforaminal approach and, if this approach has been tempted, the surgeon needs to change in order to be able to perform the operation. Anyway, as we mentioned, the majority of the surgeons prefer to reach the L5-S1 disc space by a direct midline approach and the patient under general anaesthesia.

The most important advantage of the endoscopic spinal surgery is represented by a minimally invasive approach with a minimal disruption of the normal anatomy. Also the transforaminal approach keeps the post-operative fibrosis on a minimum and make a re-do surgery easiest and less dangerous.

Among the risk and drawbacks of the transforaminal approach we must remind the damage to the nerve root, while, for the midline approach, the major risk is represented by a dural tear (the rate is similar to that one of the classical procedure). Common to all the endoscopic spinal procedures is a long and hard learning curve and consequently a long training period that can be frustrating [4]. Particularly at the beginning a simple operation can last considerably longer if compared with the same procedure done in a classical way (under general anaesthesia and with the operating microscope) and, if performed under local anaesthesia and mild sedation, can became stressful for the patient.

Eventually it is important to remind the cost related to the entire instrumentation.

Table 1 summarizes advantages and drawbacks of lumbar endoscopic discectomy

Advantages	Drawbacks
Good preservation of the normal anatomy	Nerve damage in the transforaminal approach and dural tear in the midline approach
Reduction in post-operative pain	Long and difficult learning curve
Reduction in post-operative fibrosis	Cost of the equipment
Reduced period of hospitalization	

Table 1. Advantages and drawbacks of lumbar endoscopic discectomy

The increase of the age of the population and consequently the increase of the co-morbidity with sometimes unacceptable risks for the general anaesthesia has pushed all the health personnel to find alternatives to the latter, in particular in performing spinal procedures for the most simple pathologies (disc prolapse and stenosis).

In the past many publications have stressed the possibility and opportunity to use local and regional anaesthesia for some easiest procedures, e.g. lumbar microdiscectomy and decompressive laminectomy [7, 8, 10, 11, 12]. Despite this, in the vast majority of centers these procedures are still carried out under general anaesthesia, with the patient in a prone or genu-pectoral position.

General anaesthesia has got a widespread consent and it is used routinely. It is the preferred option for anaesthesiologists because it allows an easier monitoring of vital parameters in a prone position; it is supported by surgeons because it allows extra time for surgery without problems (also useful for teaching purposes). Last but not least, patients prefer general anaesthesia since they can avoid the anxiety linked to the awareness of undergoing a surgical operation and the fear of pain [10, 12]. Nevertheless, the advantages of general anaesthesia have often outweighed its drawbacks. On this regard, we have to keep in mind potential pulmonary complications, injuries from nervous compression during the patient positioning, post-operative nausea and vomiting and extension of the operative time related to patient awaking and recovery.

In the past different publications have shown the results coming from the use of local anaesthesia for laminectomy surgery and in many occasions these publications have established that, on a particular class of selected patients (generally elderly patients with an important premorbid history), this procedure can be suitable and can offer a valid alternative to the general anaesthesia [7, 8].

The practice of the local anaesthesia for spinal surgery is not new. Traditionally, cervical osteotomies in patients with severe ankylosing spondylitis were managed in this way, mainly because they were difficult to intubate.

The use of local anaesthesia has also been previously reported in fit and healthy patients undergoing cervical laminectomy. The technique was advocated in these patients, in part, to allow neuro-monitoring during surgery. Later, other authors presented a serie of patients, with significant premorbid pathology, undergoing cervical, thoracic or lumbar decompressive laminectomy under local anaesthesia. The authors arrived to the conclusion that local anaesthesia can be very successful with minimal complications. Unfortunately the most important side effect was the pain experienced by the patient in particular during the stripping of the paravertebral muscles (a consistent finding in many patients, very difficult to manage) and not a satisfactory solution to this problem was found, except great care handling of the tissues and a well targeted infiltration of the local anaesthetic [7]. Clearly such drawback happens when the procedure is performed in the classical way that envisages the stripping of the paravertebral muscles bilaterally. It is also important to underline that this technique is only appropriate if performed by a skilled surgeon, as the patients became uniformly restless if required to lie still for, on average, more than 90 min [7].

For the reasons just mentioned, the only use of the local anaesthesia is generally not accepted and, if not contraindicated, some intravenous sedation is also administered.

As the patient is ready, the operation can also be carried out, according to the surgeon's experience, by percutaneous techniques or by endoscopic techniques whose skin incisions are often less than 1 cm long (the classical techniques generally require skin incisions 4-6 cm long). In this sense, it is evident that the percutaneous and endoscopic techniques carried out under local anaesthesia and mild sedation are able to combine all the aims that we have mentioned at the beginning of this chapter.

Indications for the use of the local anaesthesia with mild sedation can be summarized as follow: 1) Patient ability to cope with a "stressful situation". 2) Severe premorbid conditions (cardiovascular and pulmonary diseases) which may represent a significant risk for general anaesthesia. 3) No allergy toward local anaesthetics. 4) A skilled surgeon.

Table 2 summarizes indications, advantages and drawbacks of local anaesthesia for decompressive laminectomy.

Indications	Advantages	Drawbacks
Severe pre-morbid conditions (cardiovascular and pulmonary diseases)	None of risks related to the general anaesthesia	Pain related to the handling of the paravertebral muscles
Patient able to cope with a stressful situation	Possibility to discharge the patient the same day of the operation	Need of a skilled surgeon

Table 2. Indications, advantages and drawbacks of local anaesthesia for decompressive laminectomy

A valid alternative to the local anaesthesia, generally more effective in the pain control, is the injection of anaesthetic agents to create a regional block.

Under this prospective two different techniques have been developed: spinal anaesthesia and epidural anaesthesia. These techniques are erroneously considered both as the same technique and sometimes the terms are used as synonymous. Actually these two techniques are very different and currently the epidural anaesthesia is the most used.

Unlike the epidural anaesthesia, spinal anaesthesia can be used only for lumbar cases. Indeed, while epidural anaesthesia virtually can be also used for the cervical and thoracic spine, spinal anaesthesia (in consideration of the injection of anaesthetic agents in the subarachnoid space) has got the evident limit to its application to the lumbar segment in order to avoid a depression of the respiratory muscles and a dangerous bradycardia related to a sympathetic block.

To understand better the difference between these two methods it is useful to make some brief outline on the anatomy of the spine (Fig 4).

The epidural space is that potential space included between the dura and the periosteum lining the vertebral canal and it extends from the foramen magnum to the sacral hiatus. The nerve roots in their dural covering pass across this potential space to reach the intervertebral foramen where they form the segmental nerves. Anteriorly, the epidural space is bordered by the posterior longitudinal ligament covering the vertebral bodies and the intervertebral discs. Laterally, it is bordered by the periosteum of the vertebral pedicles and the intervertebral foraminae and posteriorly is bordered by the periosteum of the anterior surface of the laminae and articular processes, the periosteum of the root of the spines and the interlaminar spaces filled by the ligamentum flavum. The epidural space contains venous plexuses and fatty tissue.

The subarachnoid space is the space containing the anterior and posterior nerve roots and the CSF which is in continuity with the CSF contained in the ventricles and in the cerebral cisterns. Below the level between L1 and L2 the spinal cord ends and all the nerve roots take a configuration that resembles an cauda equina. All these nerve roots are responsible for the motility and sensation of the lower limbs and for the sphincters' control.

Before describing in details both the procedures, the indications, the contraindications (related to the selection of the appropriate patient) and the risks are outlined.

As for the local anaesthesia, for the spinal anaesthesia and epidural anaesthesia some criteria also need to be fulfilled in the patient selection. These criteria can be summarized in the following points: consented and cooperative patient; no coagulopathy or therapeutic antico-

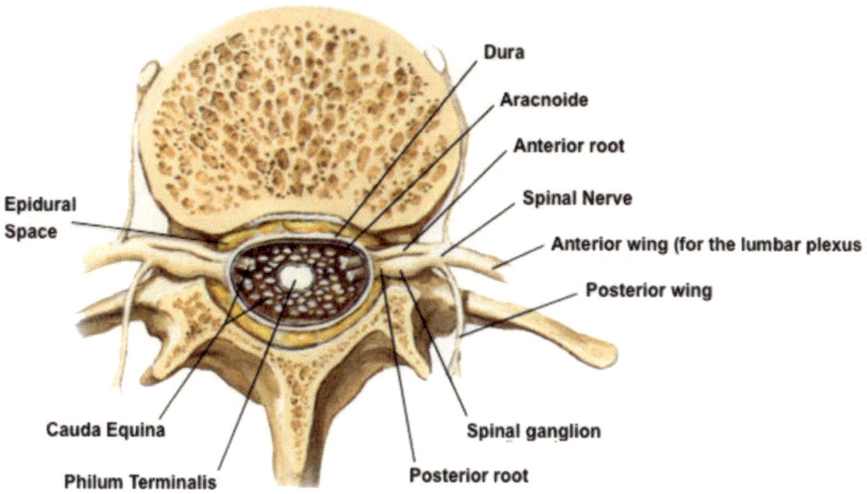

Figure 4. Axial view of the lumbar canal

agulation; no anatomical abnormalities of the spine; no allergy to anaesthetic medications; no skin infection at injection site; no hypovolaemia or fixed cardiac output states (additive risks with sympathetic block); no intracranial hypertension (risks of brain stem herniation in particular with the spinal anaesthesia) [9, 10].

Both these procedures must be performed in a work area that is equipped for airway management and resuscitation. Indeed, serious complications may occur with epidural anaesthesia and facilities for resuscitation should always be available whenever epidural or spinal anaesthesia are performed [9].

Starting with the description of the epidural anaesthesia, some standardized steps are followed: while monitoring cardiac parameters (EKG, hearth rate, blood pressure) and respiratory parameters (respiratory rate, pulse oximetry), some sedation is administered intravenously (generally 3 mg of midazolam) [10]. With the patient in a sitting or a lateral position, an intervertebral space is identified, generally two spaces above the space interested in surgery. The skin is prepared with alcohol or iodine-containing solutions and draped in a sterile fashion (the operator should take full sterile precautions, including gown, mask and gloves). Modern epidural kits are usually disposable and packed in a sterile fashion. In this sterile kit an epidural needle (17 Ga.x3-7/8"TW) is included as well as an epidural catheter that is designed to pass through the lumen of the epidural needle. A filter is also used to prevent the inadvertent injection of particulate matter into the epidural space, and as a bacterial filter. After injecting some local anaesthesia (5 mL of 2% lidocaine), the epidural needle is introduced on the midline and the epidural space is identified. To identify this space, different techniques have been developed over the years, but currently most practitioners use a syringe to identify a loss of resistance when pressure is applied to the plunger [9]. Some authors use saline in the syringe while others use air. These two methods are broadly similar, with some mild differences in the way the syringe is advanced and the epidural space entered.

Other techniques to identify the epidural space have been used in the past, e.g. the "hanging drop technique". With this technique, a drop of saline is placed at the hub of the needle and the needle (without syringe) is advanced. The epidural space is identified when the drop is "sucked" into the needle by the negative pressure characteristic of the epidural space.

When in the epidural space the local anaesthetics can be administered.

Single shot epidurals, without the use of a catheter, is still widely used in various settings, and is effective in providing intraoperative anaesthesia and analgesia in the immediate postoperative period. The major disadvantages of single shot epidurals are: 1) The duration of postoperative analgesia is limited to the duration of action of the drug given and cannot be topped up, and 2) The risks involved in injecting a full anaesthetic dose of local anaesthetics into the epidural space without a test dose and without the ability to give slow increments. This means that the risks of inadvertent high block, total spinal block and local anaesthetic toxicity are much greater. For this reason many authors prefer to avoid the single shot techniques.

The choice of drugs administered epidurally depends on the indication for the epidural.

Surgical anaesthesia requires heavy sensory block and usually moderate to heavy motor block. To achieve this, concentrated local anaesthetic preparations are required. The most commonly used local anaesthetics in this setting are 10-20ml of 2% lignocaine (with or without adrenaline 1:200000) or 10-20 mL of 0.5% bupivacaine. The latter has a longer duration of action, but a slower onset time, compared with lignocaine. Other authors prefers 8-10 ml (depending on patients' BMI) of 0,75% Ropivacaine. After the injection the patient is maintained in the sitting position for a further 30 minutes [10].

In the past the addition of opioids to local anaesthetic solutions gained popularity in particular because the opioids have a synergistic effect by acting directly on opioid receptors in the spinal cord. The combination of low-concentration local anaesthetic and low-concentration mixtures of opioids, administered by slow infusion rather than as intermittent boluses, has, in particular, been shown to be very effective in the management of postoperative pain.

The amount of opioid should be reduced where there is an increased risk of respiratory depression, i.e. the elderly or in patients with significant chronic obstructive airway disease.

Caution should be exercised when morphine is administered epidurally, as it is associated with delayed respiratory depression. This is thought to be as a result of its low lipid solubility, which means that instead of binding to opioid receptors in the spinal cord, some of the drug remains in solution in the CSF, and the circulation of CSF transports the remaining drug to the brainstem where it acts on the respiratory centre. This may occur many hours (up to 24 hours) after morphine has been administered epidurally.

Among the major risks and complications of epidural anaesthesia we must remind hypotension, a high spinal block, local anaesthesia toxicity and the total spinal block [9-12].

Hypotension is the commonest side effect of successful therapeutic blockade for procedures above the umbilicus. Vasodilatation of resistance and capacitance vessels occurs, causing relative hypovolaemia and tachycardia, with a resultant drop in blood pressure. This is

http://dx.doi.org/10.5772/58749

exacerbated by blockade of the sympathetic nerve to the adrenal glands, so preventing the release of catecholamines. If blockade is as high as T2, sympathetic supply to the heart (T2-5) is also interrupted and may lead to bradycardia. The overall result may be inadequate perfusion of vital organs and measures are required to restore the blood pressure and cardiac output, such as fluid administration and the use of vasoconstrictors. Sympathetic system arises from T1 to L2 and blockade of nerve roots below L2 is less likely to cause significant sympathetic blockade, compared with procedures requiring blockade above the umbilicus.

The inadvertent high epidural block is generally due to an excessively large dose of local anaesthetic in the epidural space. It may present with hypotension, nausea, sensory loss or paraesthesia of high thoracic or even cervical nerve roots (arms), and difficulty in breathing due to blockade of nerve supply to the intercostal muscles. These symptoms in the most severe cases may require intubation of the patient to secure the airway, while treating hypotension. If the patient has a clear airway and is breathing adequately they should be reassured and any hypotension immediately treated. Difficulty in talking (small tidal volumes due to phrenic block) and drowsiness are signs that the block is becoming excessively high and should be managed as an emergency.

Local anaesthetic toxicity can also occur as a result of an excessive dose of local anaesthetic agents in the epidural space. Even a moderate dose of local anaesthetic, if injected directly into a blood vessel, can cause toxicity. This is especially possible when an epidural catheter is inadvertently advanced into one of the many epidural veins. It is therefore vital to aspirate from the epidural catheter prior to injecting local anaesthetic. Symptoms usually follow a sequence of light-headedness, tinnitus, circumoral tingling or numbness and a feeling of anxiety or "impending doom", followed by confusion, tremor, convulsions, coma and cardiorespiratory arrest. It is important to recognize these symptoms early, and discontinue the further administration of local anaesthetic drugs. Treatment should be supportive, with the use of sedative/anticonvulsants (thiopentone, diazepam) where necessary, and cardiopulmonary resuscitation if required.

Total spinal block is a rare complication occurring when the epidural needle, or epidural catheter, is inadvertently advanced into the subarachnoid space and an "epidural dose" e.g. 10-20 mL of local anaesthetic is injected directly into the CSF. The result is a profound hypotension, apnoea, unconsciousness and dilated pupils as a result of the action of local anaesthetic on the brainstem. The use of a test dose helps in preventing most cases of total spinal block despite some cases have been described where the epidural initially appeared to be correctly sited, but subsequent top-up doses caused the symptoms of total spinal block. This has been ascribed to the migration of the epidural catheter into the subarachnoid space, although the exact mechanism is still uncertain.

Acute management of the total spinal block is based on: 1) Secure airway and administer of 100% oxygen; 2) Ventilate by facemask and intubate; 3) Treat with intravenous fluids and vasopressors; 4) Continue to ventilate until the block wears off (2-4 hours); 5) As the block recedes, the patient will begin recovering consciousness followed by breathing and then movement of the arms and finally legs.

The accidental dural puncture is usually easily recognized by the immediate loss of CSF through the epidural needle. This complication occurs in 1-2% of epidural blocks and is more related to the experience of the practitioner. It leads to a high incidence of post dural puncture headache, which is severe and associated with a number of characteristic features. The headache is typically frontal, exacerbated by movement or sitting upright, associated with photophobia, nausea and vomiting, and relieved when lying flat. The headache is thought to be due to the leakage of CSF through the puncture site. Basic measures, such as simple analgesics, caffeine, bed rest, fluid rehydration and reassurance are indicated in the first instance, and are often sufficient to treat the headache. Where the headache is severe, or unresponsive to conservative measures, an epidural blood patch may be used to treat the headache. This procedure is effective in treating approximately 90% of post dural puncture headaches. If unsuccessful, the blood patch may be repeated, and the success rate increases to 96% on the second attempt. The blood injected into the epidural space is thought to seal the hole in the dura.

Epidural haematoma is a rare but potentially catastrophic complication of epidural anaesthesia. The epidural space is filled with a rich network of venous plexuses, and puncture of these veins, with bleeding into the confined epidural space, may lead to the rapid development of a haematoma which may lead to compression of the spinal cord, and can have disastrous consequences for the patient including paraplegia and the onset of a cauda equina syndrome. For this reason, coagulopathy or therapeutic anticoagulation with heparin or oral anticoagulants is considered an absolute contraindication to epidural blockade.

Infection is another rare but potentially serious complication. Pathogenic organisms can be introduced into the epidural space if strict asepsis is not observed during the performance of the block. The commonest pathogens are Staphylococcus aureus and Streptococci. Meningitis has been described, as has epidural abscess. In addition to the symptoms of spinal cord compression described above, the patient may exhibit signs of infection such as pyrexia and a raised white cell count.

Failure of block can occur as a result of many factors, the most important being the experience of the operator. False loss of resistance during performance of the block may lead to insertion of the epidural catheter into a different area than the epidural space. Segmental sparing occurs occasionally for reasons that are unclear, but are assumed to be the result of anatomic variations of the epidural space, so that local anaesthetic fails to spread evenly throughout the space. The result is that some nerve roots are inadequately soaked with local anaesthetic, leaving the dermatomes of these nerve roots poorly anaesthetized. Unilateral blockade occurs occasionally, and this is thought to be the result of a septated epidural space, with failure of the local anaesthetic solution to spread to one half of the epidural space. Positioning the patient on his side with the unblocked side down is sometimes successful in allowing spread of the local anaesthetic to the dependent side, giving bilateral anaesthesia.

Spinal anaesthesia is the other technique that can be used; despite currently the epidural anaesthesia is the preferred one. These two techniques have relevant differences in indications, in execution and in the related risks.

Spinal anaesthesia, as we have explained before, is used only for surgery in the caudal part of the body (genital, urinary tract, or lower body procedures)

The spinal anaesthesia involves injecting a small volume of local anaesthetics (1-3.5 mL) into the spinal space below the level at which the spinal cord ends, unlike the epidural anaesthesia that involves injecting a larger volume of local anaesthetics into the space that surrounds the spinal canal and so it may be performed in any region of the back.

The local anaesthetic agents that are used provide surgical anaesthesia for 1-3 hours. For this reason, a spinal anaesthesia can only be used when the operation will take less time.

The anesthesia is performed using a needle that is thinner than that one used in the epidural anaesthesia and the needle is advanced until the subarachnoid space is reached (the discharge of CSF is the test bench. The effect starts few minutes (5-10 minutes) after the injection while with the epidural anaesthesia it can need more than 20 minutes. Another relevant difference between the two methods is the length of the effect, between 1 and 3 hours with the spinal anaesthesia and between 3 and 5 hours with the epidural anaesthesia. Also, the spinal anaesthesia is administered as a single shot and it cannot be repeated while the epidural anaesthesia can be prolonged provided that an indwelling catheter is kept in the epidural space.

Table 3 compares epidural and spinal anaesthesia and summarizes the main differences.

The major risks related to spinal anaesthesia are represented by: spinal shock, cauda equina injury, cardiac arrest, hypothermia, epidural clot, infection (meningitis, epidural abscess), severe headache, nausea, vomiting, itching, hypotension, urinary retention [9].

	Epidural anaesthesia	**Spinal anaesthesia**
Use	All the spine	Only the lumbar level
Quantity of anaesthetic agent injected (mL)	1 – 3.5	10 - 20
Onset of effect (min)	5 - 10	"/> 20
Duration of the effect (hours)	1 - 3	3 - 5
Possibility to recall	yes	No (single shot)

Table 3. Comparison between epidural anaesthesia and spinal anaesthesia

In particular with reference to the epidural anesthesia, many publications [10-18] in the past have showed that this technique is as safe and effective as general anesthesia and at the same time it allows the reduction of surgical and anaesthetic timing and the risks related to the general anaesthesia. Reduction of anaesthesia time, evidently, is linked to the elimination of the patient awaking phase, as it occurs after general anaesthesia and of the patient's recovery (post-op monitoring period).

Reduction of surgical time seems mainly related to an easier positioning of the patient and to a reduction of the intra-operative bleeding. Generally the position used during the spinal anaesthesia is the lateral decubitus (or in some occasions the sitting position), while, when a general anaesthesia is used, a prone position is preferred.

The lateral or the sitting position [10], compared to the prone one, shows benefits and drawbacks. As for the benefits we include a better comfort for the patient and the possibility to simulate the "real-life" orthostatic posture during the sitting position, often considered responsible for the onset or worsening of symptoms (this way it is possible to reveal some borderline situations, where nerve root impingement takes place only in the upright posture) (Fig. 5).

Also among the advantages of the lateral and the sitting position we must remind a "cleaner" operative field, since gravity will keep it "blood-free". This latter effect, essentially, is the result of multiple determinants: first of all, the sympatholytic effects of anaesthetic drugs used for epidural anaesthesia that are responsible for a vasodilation and a light hypotension. In addition, we must also consider the lack of increase of intrathoracic pressure, opposite to what happens for patients under general anesthesia. The lack of an upsurge of intrathoracic pressure, furthermore reinforced by not using the prone position, leads to a decreased tension in the prevertebral epidural venous plexus [15].

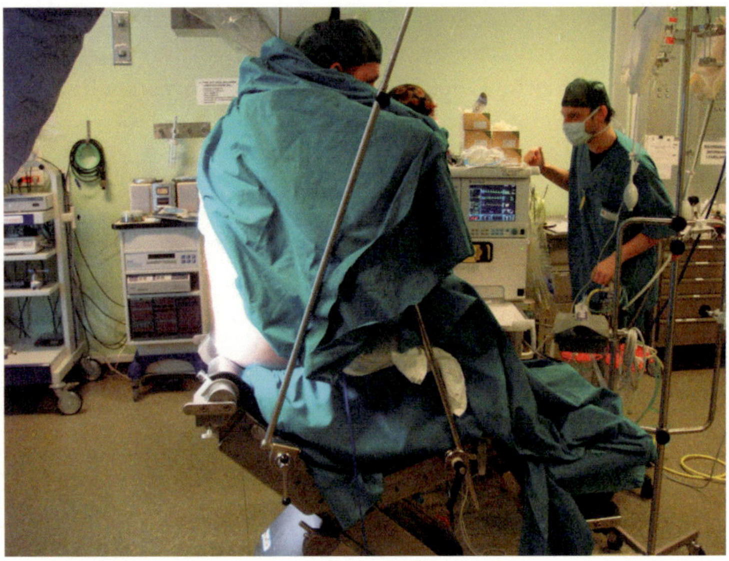

Figure 5. Patient in a sitting position on a dedicated chair

All of these mechanisms are responsible for a reduction of intraoperative bleeding, which, by speeding up the surgical procedure, allows altogether the reduction of the surgical time.

Drawbacks of the lateral and the sitting position are first of all some discomfort for the surgeon who has to work with outstretched arms (even though seated) and with the operative microscope set in a position quite similar as used for the posterior fossa surgery. This disadvantage, however, is mitigated by the shorter operating time. Surely, the most worrying drawback of the sitting position, that at the same time could be source of dangerous complications, is the possibility of a dural tear leading to CSF leak. Obviously, where a small dural tear can have no effects, a larger one could cause an important and sudden CSF leak, with a consequent risk of intracranial subdural hematomas or brain herniation syndromes. This is the reason why it is important to select the patients, by avoiding those with some risk factors (e.g.: previous surgery on the involved disc space, presence of scar tissue involving the dura, radiation therapy on the lumbar spine, etc) that could be responsible for a dural weakening [10].

In the assessment on the validity of epidural anaesthesia, some authors reported a satisfactory analgesia level reached in almost 90% of the patients undergone to epidural anaesthesia and often the only pain sensation the patient reported was a ''feeling of pressing'' [10].

Under this perspective, two more factors need to be considered: the urinary retention and the pain-free period after surgery. In the past, urinary retention was typically considered a side effect of spinal anaesthesia as compared to general anaesthesia but, in the last publications, this complication has not been showed. As observed by some authors, it is possible that at present this different trend has to be correlated to the "no use" of opioids during the induction of the epidural anaesthesia [15, 19].

The pain-free time extension after epidural anaesthesia [14,15] is harder to explain. It is likely that protopathic nervous fibers (Aδ and C), responsible for pain transmission, are more susceptible to medication used for spinal anaesthesia and resume their function more slowly than motor and epicritic sensation fibers.

Generally, the incidence of post-operative nausea or vomiting in patients who undergo spinal anaesthesia is considerably lower if compared with patients who undergo general anaesthesia, where these side effects can last for over 24 hours (leading to a longer hospital stay).

Some authors reported a slight difficulty in the placement of the muscle retractor related to the lack of a proper muscle relaxation. This led the surgeons to increase mildly (roughly 1 cm) the length of the skin incision.

In conclusion, in the current medical environment, where high medical standards have to meet lower costs, the trend is to go for surgical procedures that allow the surgeons to reach the same results with minimally invasive techniques and reducing the hospitalization time.

Under this perspective, spinal and epidural anaesthesia have gained a significant role, by allowing a reduction in anesthetic and surgical timing, in anaesthetic complications and consequently in hospital length of stay.

Despite, as usual, the right selection of the patient remains a fundamental factor to reach an optimal result, we believe that, in a near future, there will be the possibility to use these techniques to perform this type of surgery to a such an extent that they will supersede the classical techniques and will allow to manage the patient on a day-surgery basis.

Author details

Nicola Nicassio* and Irfan Malik

*Address all correspondence to: nicknave@yahoo.it

Neurosurgery Department, King's College Hospital, London, UK

References

[1] Nellensteijn J, Ostelo R, BartelsR, Peul W, Van Royen B, Van Tulder M. Transforaminal endoscopic surgery for symptomatic lumbar disc herniations: a systematic review of the literature. Eur Spine J. 2010;19:181-204.

[2] Tzaan WC Anterior percutaneous endoscopic cervical discectomy for cervical intervertebral disc herniation: outcome, complications, and technique. J Spina Disord Tech. 2011 Oct; 24(7): 421-431.

[3] Yao N, Wang C, Wang W, Wang L. Full-endoscopic technique for anterior cervical discectomy and interbody fusion: 5-year follow-up results of 67 cases. Eur Spine J. 2011 Jun;20(6):899-904.

[4] Wang H, Huang B, Li C, Zhang Z, Wang J, Zheng W, Zhou Y. Learning curve for percutaneous endoscopic lumbar discectomy depending on the surgeon's training level of minimally invasive spine surgery. Clin Neurol Neurosurg. 2013 Oct;115(10): 1987-91.

[5] Choi I, Ahn JO, So WS, Lee SJ, Choi IJ, Kim H Exiting root injury in transforaminal endoscopic discectomy: preoperative image considerations for safety. Eur Spine J. 2013 Jun 11.

[6] Chen ZG, Fu Q Percutaneous transforaminal endoscopic discectomy through different approaches for lumbar disc herniation. Zhongguo Gu Shang. 2012 Dec;25(12): 1057-60. Review. Chinese

[7] Ames.W.A., Songhurst L., Gullan R.W. Local anaesthesia for laminectomy surgery. British Journal of Neurosurgery 1999;13(6):598± 600

[8] Nygaard OP, Romner B, Thoner J, Due-Tonnessen B. Local anesthesia in posterior cervical surgery. Anestesiology 1997; 86:242± 3

[9] Dr Leon Visser Epidural Anaesthesia-Update in Anesthesia Issue 13 (2001) Article 11: page 1-4

[10] Nicassio N, Bobicchio P, Umari M, Tacconi L Lumbar microdiscectomy under epidural anaesthesia with the patient in a sitting position: A prospective study J Clin Neurosci. 2010 Dec;17(12):1537-40.

[11] Sadrolsadat SH, Mahdavi AR, Moharari RS, et al. A prospective randomized trial comparing the technique of spinal and general anesthesia for lumbar disk surgery: a study of 100 cases. Surg Neurol 2009;71:60–5

[12] Smrcka M, Baudysová O, Jurán V, et al. Lumbar disc surgery in regional anaesthesia–40 years of experience. Acta Neurochir (Wien) 2001;143:377–81

[13] Papadopoulos EC, Girardi FP, Sama A, et al. Lumbar microdiscectomy under epidural anesthesia: a comparison study. Spine J 2006;6:561–4.

[14] McLain RF, Kalfas I, Bell GR, et al. Comparison of spinal and general anesthesia in lumbar laminectomy surgery: a case-controlled analysis of 400 patients. J Neurosurg Spine 2005;2:17–22.

[15] McLain RF, Tetzlaff JE, Bell GR, et al. Microdiscectomy: spinal anesthesia offers optimal results in general patient population. J Surg Orthop Adv 2007;16:5–11

[16] Demirel CB, Kalayci M, Ozkocak I, et al. A prospective randomized study comparing perioperative outcome variables after epidural or general anesthesia for lumbar disc surgery. J Neurosurg Anesthesiol 2003;15:185–92

[17] Zou J, Yang H, Miyazaki M, et al. Dynamic bulging of intervertebral discs in the degenerative lumbar spine. Spine 2009;34:2545–50

[18] McLain RF, Bell GR, Kalfas I, et al. Complications associated with lumbar laminectomy: a comparison of spinal versus general anesthesia. Spine 2004;29:2542–7

[19] Koebbe CJ, Maroon JC, Abla A, et al. Lumbar microdiscectomy: a historical perspective and current technical considerations. Neurosurg Focus 2002;13:1–6.

Chapter 2

Spinal Anesthesia for Lower Level Spine Surgery

W. Scott Jellish and Steven Edelstein

Additional information is available at the end of the chapter

http://dx.doi.org/10.5772/58752

1. Introduction

Lumbar discectomy is the most commonly performed spinal operation in the United States with more than half a million procedures performed annually. In addition, spinal anesthesia for surgical analgesia in these procedures has been established as an accepted technique for many years. With the refinement in surgical technique for lumbar discectomy, that has now made the procedure relatively non-invasive, spinal anesthesia plays an even more important role.

The original laminectomy and discectomy was performed by Mixter and Barr in 1934 [1]. Most surgeons perform a modified microdiscectomy originally described by Williams [2]. With the use of high-powered microscopes, the anatomy is better visualized and incisions are much smaller with less tissue and bone disruption. There are alterations to the standard microdiscectomy including laser disc removal, endoscopic discectomy and intradiscal electrothermal treatment. However, the microdiscectomy remains the procedure with the highest success rate. Lumbar laminectomy or discectomy is performed with the patient in the prone or lateral decubitus position. A midline paramedian incision is created and the lumbodorsal fascia is incised. Periosteal dissection exposes the laminae that are removed as necessary to provide access to the thecal sac and nerve roots. The nerve roots are retraced medially to expose the posterior longitudinal ligament that covers the intervertebral discs. The discectomy is performed by incising the ligament and removing disc material with a forceps. The laminar resection can also be extended to provide canal decompression in cases of spinal stenosis.

It is important to note that the lumbar spine has the largest vertebral bodies and bears the greatest weight. The center of gravity of the body is approximately 1 cm behind the sacral promontory that, in turn, places the entire weight of the body directly on $L_{4\text{-}5}$ and $L_{5\text{-}S1}$. With aging, the discs tend to become less fluid and more fibrocartilagenous, with little difference between nucleus and annulus. The discs are subject to pathologic changes that may lead to herniation of the nucleus pulposus and cause compression of the neural elements.

Subsequent removal of the disc or lamina with the assistance of loops or microscopes typically has a surgical duration of approximately two hours. As such, this has made spinal anesthesia an attractive choice for the anesthetic technique in these patients. This chapter will review the evidence supporting the utilization of this technique as well as the possible risks associated with neuraxial anesthesia and prone positioning.

2. Technique of spinal anesthesia for spine surgery

Briefly, once a decision has been made to proceed with spinal anesthesia several items must be performed in order to have a successful outcome. Knowing the level of surgical anesthesia required is extremely important since this will determine whether the patient can comfortably undergo the procedure and avoid the hemodynamic consequences of surgical stimulation. Of course, it is also essential that the area of coverage will provide relief from painful stimuli as well.

Anesthesia levels for lumbar surgery can be easily achieved with hyperbaric or isobaric local anesthetics. Typically, for L1-L5 surgery a dermatomal sensory level of at least T6-T8 will be required. Though this is higher than the level of the operative site, the higher level will allow for the surgery to take place and, depending on the local anesthetic selected, allow for a slow regression of surgical anesthesia coverage. In most instances, the patient is placed in the full prone position. The prone knee chest position and the horizontal side position have also been used. These positions are of importance since the spread of local anesthetic may be different depending on this position and also the baricity of the local anesthetic solution. After placing the spinal, the patient should be positioned supine with the level allowed to set before final positioning is achieved.

Bupivacaine appears to be the agent of choice since it provides adequate duration of coverage in comparison to other agents such as lidocaine. If lidocaine is selected, it is conceivable that regression of sensory coverage could occur shortly after positioning and draping of the patient. In addition, some practitioners will also select additives to the local anesthetic though the risk/benefits of these will be discussed later. A variety of agents have been used in lumbar surgery, all with varying degrees of success including opioids, epinephrine, phenylephrine, neostigmine and clonidine. Final selection of any and all additives will depend on the clinical situation and the physical status of the patient.

In most instances, the patient will have the spinal anesthetic placed prior to prone positioning. Usually the patient will be administered 400-600 ml of a balanced salt solution to expand intravascular volume prior to spinal placement. The preference for placement of the spinal block for many practitioners is to place the patient in the seated position. The seated position allows for better delineation of the overall spinal anatomy and helps to ascertain the midline, especially in larger individuals. In some instances, the patient can be placed in the lateral decubitus position for spinal placement. The back is prepped and draped in a sterile fashion and the best interspace, either L2-3, 3-4 or 4-5, is identified and 2-4 ml of 2% lidocaine is injected to anesthetize the area where the spinal needle will be inserted. Most practitioners will use a 24g or 25g pencil-point spinal needle placed through an introducer and advanced until free flow of CSF is observed from the hub of the needle. The spinal anesthetic can also be accomplished with the use of a 22 gauge Quincke needle. Once subarachnoid placement is confirmed, either 2-3 ml of 0.5% plain bupivacaine or 1.5-2 ml of 0.75% hyperbaric bupivacaine is injected into the subarachnoid space. The patient is returned to the supine position, and once a T8-10 level is obtained, the patient is rolled into the prone position and either placed on chest rolls, a Wilson or Andrews frame and allowed to self position their upper body for comfort.

3. Baricity issues

There has been some controversy over the preferred baricity of the local anesthetic for spinal anesthesia in lumbar surgery. Jellish, et al, [3] in their prospective study effectively utilized hyperbaric bupivacaine 0.75% with dextrose 8.5% to achieve levels of T6-T10. The study patients were required to stay supine after placement of the local anesthetic for approximately 10 minutes to fix the spinal level. Fixation of a hyperbaric spinal is required since typically the patients are placed in prone position. This is of particular importance given the fact that there are times when the head-down position is transiently performed as the patient is positioned on a frame or in knee-chest position.

If a hyperbaric solution is selected and adequate time for fixation has not been performed, the solution could track cephalad and lead to a higher level than what is required. This is also accentuated since the frame and/or knee-chest position required for the surgery eliminates the lordotic curves of the spine. The fixation of a hyperbaric spinal occurs when the solution is taken up by the spinal tissue and blood, especially the dextrose solution. This results in a change in solution from hyperbaric to isobaric and subsequent positioning has little to no effect [4].

Baricity of the spinal anesthetic has also been shown to affect both the quality of the anesthetic and the level of the block. Isobaric procaine/tetracaine spinal anesthesia has the same success profile with minimal complication compared to general anesthesia for spine surgery [5]. If the sensory level is adequate and ventilation is not impaired by a high block, spinal anesthesia provides good surgical conditions for spine surgery. Subjective dyspnea associated with a high spinal level may be accentuated with the patient in the prone position. Some clinicians believe isobaric spinal anesthetics could be the best choice because the dense low thoracic block may be routinely achieved with minimal hemodynamic consequences. Also, the effect of the isobaric agent is not affected by other factors like gravity or prolonged position. As such, patients that are placed in the knee chest position can be turned prone immediately after placement of the spinal as opposed to wait times of 10 minutes or longer for the block to set with a hyperbaric technique.

Plain isobaric bupivacaine was compared to hyperbaric bupivacaine to determine quality of block and cephalad spread in patients undergoing spinal surgery [6]. A 3 mL solution of isobaric 0.5% bupivacaine was administered to one group and 2ml of 0.75% bupivacaine was administered to the second group. All injections were performed within 5 seconds with the needle bevel facing cephalad. After turning supine for 10 minutes, the patients were turned prone to begin surgery. Time of onset for sensory and motor block was more rapid with hyperbaric bupivacaine. In addition, the final level achieved was higher with hyperbaric bupivacaine, compared to isobaric solution. Maximum heart rate change was similar in both groups but maximum blood pressure change was greater with the hyperbaric solution and this required a greater need for blood pressure and heart rate treatments. The dependent movement of hyperbaric solutions, and the level of the block achieved was always several denervations higher than the equivalent dose of isobaric solution. Even though sensory block is higher with hyperbaric local anesthetics, sympathetic block could be even higher. This explains the alteration in blood pressure observed with hyperbaric spinal anesthesia that is accentuated by turning prone. Thus, when using hyperbaric bupivacaine, meticulous determination of block level must be made before positioning the patient to avoid hypotension and bradycardia.

More breakthrough pain during spinal surgery has been noted with hyperbaric bupivacaine solutions compared to isobaric. This is thought to be due to the superiority of plain bupivacaine in suppressing slow conducting repetitive stimuli that is characteristic of low back pain [7].

Rung and colleagues [8] have suggested the utilization of isobaric bupivacaine 0.5% for providing adequate anesthesia. The group felt that the isobaric nature of the medication would help avoid the issues regarding positioning and unwanted rises in anesthetic levels. In addition, they also felt that the utilization of isobaric agents would speed the procedure since the patient could first be placed in prone position and then have the anesthetic administered. This would decrease the amount of time required for preparation and speed the onset of surgery.

Another study examined the use of 15 mg of 0.5% plain bupivacaine injected at the $L_{2\text{-}3}$ interspace and either placing the patient in the prone knee chest position before placement of the spinal or after spinal placement positioning the patient supine and allowing the spinal level to be obtained before positioning prone. [9] The mean drop in systolic blood pressure was 30 mmHg in prepositioned patients compared to 13 mmHg with spinal placed before positioning. More ephedrine was needed when the spinal was placed post positioning to maintain blood pressure compared to the patients who had the block placed in the horizontal side position. This same knee chest group of patients also needed more atropine or glycopyrrolate to maintain heart rate. The investigators believed that placing the spinal block in the lateral horizontal position and allowing the patient to lie supine for 20 minutes produced less hypotension and bradycardia when compared to patients who had the block placed in the prone knee chest position because these patients had more time to accommodate for vasodilation of the lower limbs. The controversy over the ideal baricity has not been settled and either agent may be appropriate for the procedure.

Typically during the insertion of the spinal anesthetic a pencil-point needle such as a Whitacre is used versus the standard cutting Quincke type. Obviously this is utilized to avoid undue trauma to the dura via the cutting needle and causing a potential dural tear that could interfere with surgery (cerebral spinal fluid (CSF) in the field) as well as lead to postdural puncture headaches. In addition, other studies suggest that the pencil-point needles lead to a local inflammatory response that help with rapid dural closure [10].

The appropriate level of needle insertion will obviously be determined by the procedure and what disc is affected. There have been concerns about the utilization of spinal anesthesia in patients with pre-existing spinal disease; however in a report by Hebl et al., [11] it was felt that the history of spinal surgery did not increase the risk of technical complications or block success, but did make placement potentially more difficult. The group felt that midline or lateral approach may be especially difficult if there were bone grafting or posterior fusions since success would only occur if the block was performed at areas that were unfused.

Prone (for isobaric only), sitting or lateral approaches for spinal anesthesia insertion have all been described, however is must be kept in mind that ultimately the spinal should be placed above the level of any lumbar stenosis (and below the level of the cord) since very tight stenotic lesions may affect spread of local anesthetic [12].

4. Additional issues regarding agent selection

Currently procaine, lidocaine, mepivacaine, tetracaine, ropivacaine, levobupivacaine, bupivacaine are all approved in the US for intrathecal use. As mentioned previously, bupivacaine is typically the choice of agent due to its duration of action. Ropivacaine and L-bupivacaine (S-enantiomer of bupivacaine) have a less cardiotoxic profile compared to bupivacaine; however, the overall volume utilized in spinal anesthesia is so small that this is of little concern. Tetracaine, which is an ester-based local anesthetic may also be utilized and may be in prepared in isobaric, hypobaric or hyperbaric solutions. Typically, because fixation for tetracaine takes a long time, it is not routinely utilized.

Lidocaine has a long history of safe use, but its association with transient neurologic symptoms (TNS) would make it a potentially poor choice for lumbar spine surgery. TNS, initially described in 1993[13] presents with the onset of back and leg pain post-procedure. It has been associated with positioning and can be found with all local anesthetics, but has been reported most frequently with lidocaine. Still there is no definitive proof that the local anesthetics are the source for TNS and some studies have strongly encouraged the discontinuation of this term to avoid linking the previous clinical symptoms with the use of lidocaine [14].

It is well known that determinants for level of spinal analgesia depend on the dosage administered as well as the baricity [15]. The total dose of bupivacaine administered is very important since the concentration of the medication changes after mixing with the CSF and the change in concentration has on the quality or level of the spinal anesthesia [16]. In addition, other studies have determined that there is non-homogenous spread of local anesthetics in the CSF

[4]. Typically there is an epicenter of local anesthetic concentration and subsequent spread away from the site with decreasing levels of local. The decreased concentration at these sites leads to a variation in uptake of the anesthetic in the level of the cord.

5. Additives

As with most spinal anesthetics, there may be the desire to place additives to enhance the quality of the block utilized for lumbar surgery. Opioids, vasoconstrictors, alpha-2 agonists and neostigmine [17] have all been described and each has associated risk and benefits. Opioids tend to work synergistically with local anesthetics and are known to enhance the quality of the block. However, these agents are also associated with urinary retention (a controversy that will be discussed later). Concern regarding the addition of vasopressors and spinal blood flow is unfounded and their overall mechanism of action is unclear and inconsistent depending on the agent chosen [18].

Clonidine, an alpha-2 agonist, has been utilized frequently in spinal surgery. It is known to block the motor and sensory affects associated with tetracaine, but sensory affects are much longer. The proposed mechanism is related to the vasoconstrictive properties and the antinociception associated with adrenergic stimulation and activation of the descending noradrenergic pathways [18, 19]. Other investigators noted that patients who underwent spinal surgery and received 150mg of clonidine epidurally displayed lower postanesthesia care unit pain scores and less demand for analgesics as well as improved postoperative hemodynamics [20]. These results were confirmed in a study by Farmery and Wilson-MacDonald who found that utilization of an epidural catheter with clonidine after spinal surgery (under general anesthesia) led to profound and prolonged postoperative pain relief along with a reduction in postoperative nausea and vomiting [21]. The use of clonidine will be discussed further in the section regarding pain control.

6. Benefits

Some of the benefits of performing spinal anesthesia for lumbar surgery include a perceived decrease in blood loss, lower rates of thromboembolism, less hypertension or tachycardia, and better postoperative pain control. In addition, during spinal anesthesia, the patient is only mildly sedated with a benzodiazepine or propofol. This allows for a more reliably assessment of potential positioning issues that will be discussed later.

7. Blood loss

It has been observed that there is a perception of less surgical blood loss associated with cases performed under spinal anesthesia. Preload is markedly reduced during spinal anesthesia and there is a resultant drop in mean arterial pressure (MAP). This reduction will produce a decrease in vertebral interosseous pressure during neuraxial anesthesia which may lead to reduced blood pressure within the bone itself, considered the main source of bleeding during posterior lumbar spine surgery [22]. The mechanism in which spinal anesthesia may reduce blood loss may possibly be related to the fact that spinal anesthesia leads to a marked reduction in the high venous pressure that occurs in response to sympathetic activity provoked by pain produced by tissue damage during surgery [23]. On the contrary, inhalational anesthesia does not totally block these sensory signals but these signals are effectively inhibited with spinal anesthesia.

Spinal anesthesia permits spontaneous ventilation during surgery that in the prone position results in lower intrathoracic pressure compared with general anesthesia using positive pressure ventilation. The avoidance of positive pressure ventilation results in less distension of the epidural veins and a reduction in intrathoracic pressure. This reduction produces a better blood return through the vena cava and less blood flow and distention of the venous plexus for better surgical exposure [24]. The diminished blood loss observed during spinal anesthesia can facilitate removal of the disc or vertebral body and result in less surgical time observed because of reduced time to affect hemostasis.

It is also worth reviewing the hemodynamic effects of spinal anesthesia since they play a significant role in the reduction of blood loss. Spinal anesthetics are known to produce a sympathetic denervation that is more profound as the level of anesthesia progresses. When a partial sympathetectomy occurs, as is routine with a well-controlled spinal, the area of tissue above the level of sympathetic denervation displays a reflex increase in sympathetic tone. This helps to compensate for the peripheral vasodilation that subsequently occurs. Arterial and arteriole beds are affected but do not maximally vasodilate due to the maintenance of autonomous tone. Thus, it is common to see a mild decrease in total peripheral vascular resistance of approximately 15-18% assuming cardiac output is maintained [4].The venous circulation, however, is profoundly affected and since, in spine surgery, the extremities lie below the level of the heart, there is a significant amount of pooling of the blood in the dependent capacitance vessels. If normovolemia is not maintained then a significant decrease in cardiac output is seen.

8. Blood pressure and coronary circulation

There have been numerous studies comparing spinal with general anesthesia, and in most instances there has been minimal intraoperative hemodynamic differences between the two techniques. In many of the comparisons, total anesthesia times were shorter with the use of spinal as compared to general anesthesia (GA) [3, 25, 26]. (Table 1) In all of these studies it was noted that mean arterial pressure and heart rate were lower in patients receiving spinal anesthesia. The incidence of bradycardia was lower in spinal anesthesia as well as the incidence of tachycardia. The observation that spinal anesthesia maintains hemodynamic stability with little effect on heart rate was noted in a recent study by Attari, et al [27]. In this study 72 patients underwent spine surgery with half assigned to general anesthesia and the other to spinal anesthesia. Statistically significant reductions in MAP and heart rate changes were noted in the spinal group. In addition there was enhanced surgeon satisfaction as well as a reduction in postoperative pain. These results were supported in another study which compared sixty patients undergoing lumbar disk surgery [28]. This group noted like Attari, that there were less episodes of tachycardia, hypertension and better postoperative pain with less nausea/vomiting in patients undergoing spinal. However, in their study, they found that surgeon satisfaction was greater in the general anesthesia group.

	Spinal	**General**
Total anesthesia time (min)	106.6±3.2	131.0±4.3*
Surgical time (min)	67.1±2.8	81.5±3.6*
Blood loss (mL)	133±13	221±32*
Intravenous fluids (mL)	1329±60	1478±79
Bradycardia	14.0%	22.9%
Hypertension	3.3%	26.2%*
Tachycardia	14.8%	21.3%
Hypotension	54.1%	57.4%
Ephedrine required	36.1%	22.9%

Numeric dara expressed as mean ± SEM

Bradycardia and hypotension=decreases in heart rate (HR) and mean arterial pressure (MAP) to less than 80% of baseline values; tachycardia and hypertension=HR and MAP greater than 120% of baseline values.

*P<0.05 versus spinal anesthesia group.

Jellish et al. Spinal vs General Anesthesia for Spinal Surgery. Anesth Analg 1996;83:559-64

Table 1. Intraoperative Data for Spinal versus Genera; Anesthesia Groups

Another recent comparative study also found the incidence of tachycardia to be higher with general anesthesia [29]. They found the incidence of bradycardia to be similar, as well as intravenous fluids and operative times. They did note a higher incidence of hypotension with spinal anesthesia compared to the other studies. This may reflect the importance of the fluid preload prior to the placement of the spinal block which was not used in that study.

Patients undergoing lumbar procedures under spinal anesthesia seemed to have similar or better hemodynamic variables than patients having the procedure under general anesthesia. Less intraoperative hypertension is noted and less tachycardia is observed with spinal anesthesia. Tetzloff, et al. [30]. using power spectral heart rate data which included low frequency, high frequency and the ratios of low/high frequency demonstrated that with spinal dermatomal levels below $T_{8,}$ the prone position resulted in a significant increase in heart rate with spinal anesthesia and a significant decrease in blood pressure with general anesthesia. Low frequency and low frequency/high frequency ratios were unchanged in the spinal anesthesia group. The preservation of low frequency heart rate variation may reflect better presentation of cardiac sympathetic activity with spinal anesthesia. Low thoracic levels of spinal anesthesia preserve the sympathetic efferent signals to the myocardium more than general anesthesia. Placing a patient in the prone position may reduce venous return and preload which is better tolerated with a spinal anesthetic.

Given the fact that many of the patients presenting for spinal surgery may have co-morbidities such as coronary artery disease, one may be concerned regarding the presence of hypotension. It has been noted that the decrease in MAP results in a significant decrease in coronary blood flow. One investigator found that there was a 48% decrease in myocardial oxygen supply during spinal anesthesia but there was also a 53% decrease in myocardial oxygen requirements [31]. There are three reasons for the decrease in myocardial oxygen requirement that include the reduction in afterload, preload and heart rate. Heart rate reduction is related to both the vagal predominance that occurs after sympathetectomy as well as the decrease in right atrial pressures and pressures in the great veins (via intrinsic chronotropic stretch receptors) which leads to bradycardia [4].

9. Pain control

Improving postoperative analgesia in spine surgery patients is also a challenge. Though many of the patients who receive spinal anesthesia for their spine procedure have reduced pain scores and analgesia requirements in the immediate postoperative period, their analgesic requirements are similar to general anesthesia patients 24 hours after surgery. Several studies comparing the two anesthetics demonstrated that patients who had spinal anesthesia had lower pain scores and analgesic requirements [3, 25, 29]. In many of the studies the lower pain scores may result from two different mechanisms. Patients who received spinal anesthesia had much lower initial pain scores than general anesthesia patients. There may be a preemptive effect in which spinal anesthesia attenuates pain by inhibiting afferent nociceptive pathways [32]. Also, since sensory recovery will lag behind motor recovery after spinal block, the patients receiving neuroaxial anesthesia likely had residual blockade even though motor function had returned.

Pain after spine procedures is a combination of musculoskeletal, usually derived from surgical trauma and neuropathy that is radiating and burning in nature and is secondary to the nerve compression or injury that required the laminectomy or discectomy. This type of pain responds poorly to opioids but has been shown to be relieved with the administration of epidural clonidine [33].

Sympathetic hyperactivity is reduced from the administration of epidural clonidine through three mechanisms. It may inhibit nociceptor neurotransmitter release in the dorsal horn and sympathetic outflow in the spinal cord intermediolateral column. In addition, it may inhibit norepinephrine release from sympathetic terminals in the periphery. Clonidine may also be absorbed into the systemic circulation where it reaches alpha 2 adrenoreceptors of the dorsal horn and provides analgesia by increasing the antinoceptive threshold of the spinal cord which activates the descending noradrenergic pathway to inhibit small diameter afferent induced substance P release [19].

The addition of epidural clonidine to spinal anesthetics for spine surgery has been found to reduce pain in patients receiving rescue analgesics to increase the time to the first rescue dose of analgesics for pain. Clonidine prolongs sensory and motor block associated with intrathecal bupivacaine [34]. Patients who received epidural clonidine along with their spinal anesthetic required their first analgesia dose 3.7 hours after surgery [20]. Another study showed that by using a small dose combination of epidural morphine and clonidine for postoperative analgesia after lumbar disc surgery reduced pain with movement after surgery[35]. These patients experienced a frequent incidence of difficult micturition not observed when epidural clonidine was administered without added opioids.

The infiltration of local anesthetics into the surgical wound has also been noted to prolong postoperative analgesia after lumbar spine surgery. The infiltration of 0.375% bupivacaine subcutaneously has been noted to produce an analgesic effect which lasted approximately 13 hours [36]. With the use of newer local anesthetics that have a timed release, this type of analgesia could be even more prolonged [37].

The success rate of the spinal anesthetic in patients with spinal pathology is also a consideration. Some practitioners have noted ineffective spread or patchy block with spinal anesthesia after previous spine surgery. There are a number of problems that could affect the spread of the local anesthetic including altered anatomy which may make placement of the spinal more difficult. Insertion of a spinal needle through the site of a fusion may be complicated by scar tissue and bone graft material. Intradural scarring commonly referred to as arachnoiditis, characterized by an inflammation of the pia arachnoid membrane surrounding the spinal cord may alter the anatomy of the subarachnoid space and limit the spread of local anesthetics [38]. Most investigators have noted a high success rate of spinal anesthesia after previous spinal surgery with failure rates of less than 1% [26].

10. Venous thromboembolism

Finally, spinal anesthesia for lumbar spine surgery also decreases the incidence of lower extremity thromboembolic complications [39]. The most likely explanation is the modulation of the hypercoagulable state that occurs after surgery. Neuraxial anesthesia with local anesthetics has been shown to enhance fibrinolytic activity, reduce antithrombin III activity to normal levels and attenuate increases in postoperative platelet activity [40].

11. Postoperative nausea

Many studies have noted a reduced incidence in postoperative nausea and vomiting. The increased need for narcotic analgesics in patients receiving GA may be a contributing factor to the higher amount of emetic symptoms with GA. In addition, anesthetic factors such as the use of N_2O (nitrous oxide) or the administration of certain pungent inhalational anesthetics could produce more nausea after surgery. The incidence of nausea and vomiting has also been demonstrated to be less with low level T-8 or bolus spinal anesthesia compared to GA because of improved gastric emptying.

12. Post-anesthesia care unit (PACU)

Hemodynamics in the PACU have been noted to be better with spinal anesthesia compared to GA. Both heart rate and blood pressure have been noted to be higher in GA patients upon admit to PACU. (Figure 1) This may be due to the increased sympathetic activity during emergence from anesthesia and possibly undertreated pain with opioids or other analgesics prior to emergence. Patients who had spinal anesthesia were much less hypertensive throughout their recovery room stay.

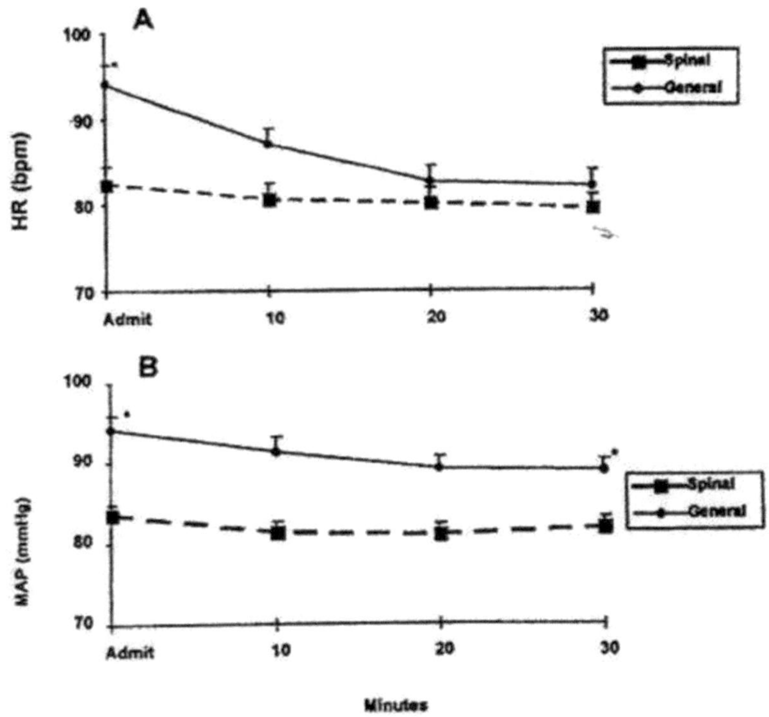

Jellish et al. Spinal vs General Anesthesia for Spine Surgery. Anesth Analg 1996;83:559-64

Figure 1. Heart rate (HR) and mean arterial pressure (MAP) values at admission (admit) and at 10, 20 and 30 min after adimission to the postanesthesia care unit (PACU). Intergroup differences in HR (A) were noted at PACU admission but did not persist through 20-min time point. Intergroup differences in MAP (B) were also observed at PACU admission and were still present 30 min after admission. *Significant difference compared to spinal group at a $P<0.001$ level.

13. Rare complications

Complications associated with spinal anesthesia for lumbar surgery have been relatively rare. There have been no reports of post-dural puncture headache even when a dural tear occurred during surgery [9].A possible explanation is that surgery near the spinal cord elicits inflammatory responses that help seal any small puncture site. In addition, the presence of small amounts of post-procedural blood may serve to seal the site similar to applying a blood patch. Other complications associated with spinal anesthesia may play a role in these lumbar cases and will be discussed further.

14. Neurological complications

In general, spinal anesthesia has a long history of safety. In the widely quoted study by Dripps and Vandam, properly performed spinal anesthesia is safe. A study which reviewed over 10,000 spinal anesthetics failed to find any major neurologic sequelae [41]. However, in a retrospective study by Hebl et al, [11], one of the major findings was that the patient population with pre-existing spinal stenosis or disk disease had an increased risk of worsening pre-existing deficits or development of new deficits after neuraxial blockade. In addition, those patients with multiple neurologic diagnoses have even higher risk. It was noted that the frequency of persistent postoperative neurologic deficits was approximately 1.1% (95% CI 0.5-2%) with prior epidemiological investigations being somewhere between 1:1000 to 1:10,000.

The group went on to propose that the neurological problems seen may have been the result of a "double-crush" phenomenon [42].In double-crush syndrome there is a pre-existing lesion (proximal) and distal to the lesion there is another compression that renders the nerve vulnerable to further injury. Neuraxial anesthesia may add insult by the additive effects of neural ischemia and local anesthetic toxicity. In spinal anesthesia, local anesthetic toxicity resulting from maldistribution and high concentrations is well known. This toxicity has resulted in cauda equina syndrome seen with microcatheters utilized for continuous spinal anesthesia [43]. Though these studies are worrisome, there have yet to be reports of neurological complications from spinal anesthesia used for lumbar spine surgery.

15. Cardiac arrest

Though it has been mentioned previously that there is less observed bradycardia during spinal anesthesia for spine surgery, there still exists the concern for profound bradyarrhythmias and cardiac arrest. In a review of studies about cardiac arrest during spinal anesthesia, investigators found an overall incidence of 0.07% (7 for every 10,000 patients) [44]. More than half were in patients under the age of thirty and this may explain the paucity of events during lumbar surgery with an older patient population. The mechanism proposed is a result of the blockade of sympathetic efferents that leads to bradyarrhythmias via vagal predominance. The presence of vagal mediated bradycardia and decreased venous return from venodilation combines to cause further issues. It is well known that right atrial pressures are decreased in low spinals (36%) and high spinals (up to %53) [45]. This decrease in preload elicits reflexes that cause severe bradycardia [46]:

- Pacemaker stretch → decrease venous return → decrease atrial stretch → decrease heart rate
- Firing of low pressure baroreceptors in the right atrium
- Bezold-Jarisch reflex

The Bezold-Jarisch reflex (BJR) is triggered by the stimulation of intracardiac mechanoreceptors that subsequently lead to bradycardia, hypotension and vasodilation [47]. According to Mackey [46] and Kinsella [48], the mechanoreceptors associated with BJR are usually triggered by distention, but when there is a decrease in venous return (as seen with prone position and spinal anesthesia), along with an increase in inotropic state (compensatory response to decreased preload), the walls of the ventricle may deform and trigger the mechanoreceptors similar to what is seen during distention. This results in a paradoxical vasodepressor response. This vasodepressor response along with the pre-existing bradycardia may lead to cardiac arrest. It is interesting to note that the BJR is also triggered by spinal anesthesia via 5-HT_3 receptors in the vagal nerve endings. The 5-HT_3 trigger can be abolished by the administration of ondansetron, an antagonist to 5-HT_3.

Risk factors identified by Pollard [44] that are associated with cardiac arrest include the following:

- Baseline heart rate <60
- ASA status I
- Use of beta blocking drugs
- Sensory level above T6
- Age <50 years
- Prolonged PR interval

Recommendations include the maintenance of preload whenever possible, followed by a step-wise escalation of pharmacological intervention starting with atropine (0.4-0.6 mg), then ephedrine (25-50 mg) and finally, if still not responsive, epinephrine (0.2-0.3 mg) intravenously.

16. Urinary retention

Urinary retention has also been associated with spinal anesthesia. However, in several studies the incidence of urinary retention was not different with spinal or general anesthesia. In most situations when spinal anesthesia is associated with urinary retention, opioids were added to the local anesthetic [49]. Subarachnoid opioids clearly increase the incidence of urinary retention, as well as respiratory depression, drowsiness and pruritis. We tend not to utilize opioids as part of the spinal anesthetic.

17. Other potential problems

17.1. Prone positioning issues

Positioning related neurologic injury has also been noted to occur more frequently during spinal surgery in the prone positioned patient [50].The most prevalent is injury to the brachial plexus. Injury to the brachial plexus is attributed to its long and superficial course in the axilla and its attachment to two firm points of fixation, the vertebrae proximally and the axillary fascia distally in the arm. The plexus also passes directly beneath the clavicle and above the first rib (Figure 2). This close proximity to freely moving bony structures makes this nerve bundle prone to stretching and compression from arm malposition. Brachial plexus injury occurs most frequently when the patient is in the prone position, especially when the arms are adducted more than 90°. In this position traction on the plexus and compression between the clavicle and first rib is responsible for the neurologic deficit. If patients are placed in the lateral decubitus position, they may be subject to brachial plexus injury from compression when the dependent arm and shoulder are positioned between the thorax and the table.

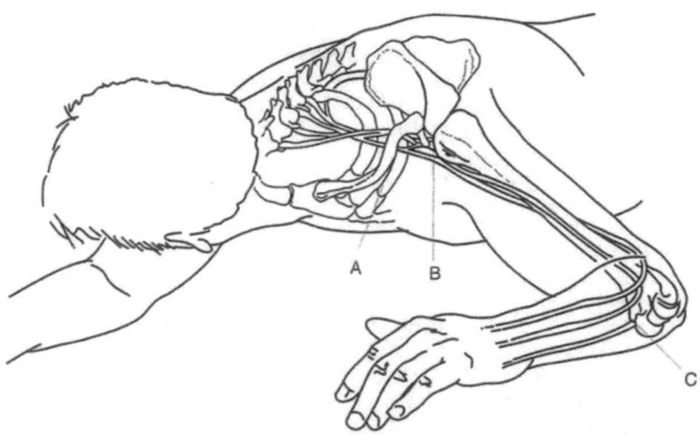

Jellish et al. Spinal Anesthesia for Spinal Surgery. Best Practices & Research. Clinical Anaesthesiology 2003;17(3): 323-334

Figure 2. Possible areas of injury to the brachial plexus: (A) neck rotation away from arm may cause stretch and compression between clavicle and first rib; (B) injury to plexus at humeral head; (C) compression or ulnar nerve in cubital tunnel.

The eyes and ears are also of concern in prone positioned patients. Pressure on the globe or hypotension, with venous congestion, could result in increased intraocular pressure and possible blindness related to ischemic injury to the optic nerves. There have been reports of increased extraocular pressure resulting from using a cushion or horseshoe head-rest to position the face [51, 52].In addition, ECG monitoring wires or oral gastric tubes, if present, could migrate under the head during prone positioning. The face could lie directly on these objects causing pressure induced ischemia to the face or eyes. These problems are avoided with the use of spinal anesthesia. The patient may be only mildly sedated and using their upper body can help to self-position with their head on a pillow or cushion. If abnormal positioning occurs, the patient will feel discomfort and alert the practitioner to the problems. They can also move their arms and head to avoid prolonged abnormal or awkward position that could produce injury.

17.2. Sedation issues

A spinal anesthetic with an awake or sedated patient who is spontaneously breathing may not be ideal for all spine surgeries. Prone positioning on different positioning systems can affect cardiac output with the possibility of a significant decrease in stroke volume and cardiac index in conjunction with the development of increased vascular and pulmonary resistance [53] (Figure 3). Patients with normal cardiac status can usually tolerate these changes. However, patients with compromised cardiac status might not be able to tolerate supine to prone positioning, especially with decreased sympathetic tone. A large drop in blood pressure or cardiac output could affect consciousness and spontaneous breathing.

Type	Picture	Chest Support	Abdomen	Pelvis	Legs
Siemens Positioning System	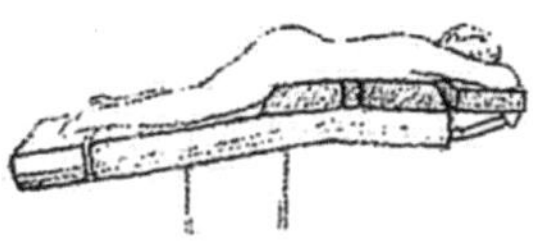	Yes	Partial compression	Supported	At heart level
Andrews Frame	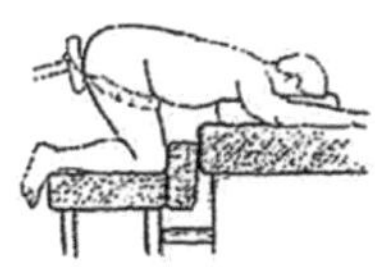	Yes	Hangs free	Partial support	Below heart
Wilson Frame	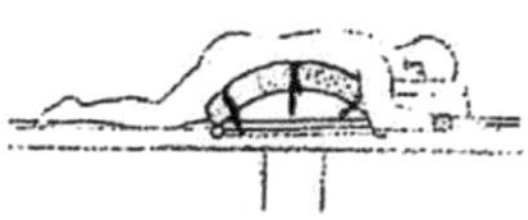	Yes	Partial compression	Partial support	Slightly below
Jackson Spine Table	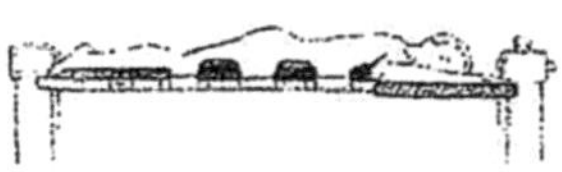	Yes	Hangs free	Supported	Supported at thigh At heart level
Longitudinal Bolster	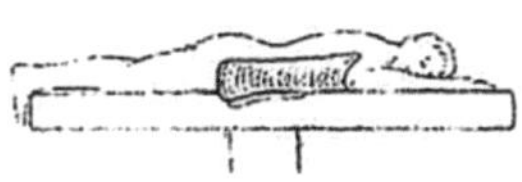	Partial	Partial compression	Partial support	At heart level

Jellish et al. Effects of Prone Positioning Systems on Hemodynamic and Cardiac Function During Lumbar Spine Surgery: An Echocardiographic Study. Spine 2006:31(12) 1388-1393

Figure 3. Description of the five different positioning systems used in this study. The type of body support each positioner provides and lower extremity position in relation to the heart are also described.

In addition, surgeries that may last more than 2-3 hours may not be conducive for spinal anesthesia. The tolerance for prone positioning on a frame in an awake or mildly sedated patient is approximately 2 hours. Patients become restless and tend to begin to adjust position in order to relieve the strain of maintaining one position for a prolonged period of time. A cooperative surgeon who can perform the procedure in a reasonable amount of time is imperative.

We also believe one to two level laminectomies or discectomies are ideal for this technique. Larger laminectomies for multi-level fusions would be too prolonged to be well tolerated in the spontaneously breathing sedated patient. Body habitus must also be considered in selecting the appropriate patient for spinal anesthesia for spine surgery. Large, obese patients with protuberant abdomens may not tolerate prone positioning well, especially if breathing spontaneously. Their ability to breathe against the restrictive effects of a large abdomen, especially if not adequately decompressed by the positioning system, could cause the patient undue anxiety and intolerance because of the inability to adequately deep breath.

18. Summary

Spinal anesthesia is an appropriate technique for lumbar spine procedures of two to three hours duration. An appropriate patient and cooperative surgeon will also facilitate the use of this anesthetic technique. The ability of the patient to self-position and guard against position related injury is of major benefit. A better postoperative experience with less pain, nausea and hemodynamic stability make this technique superior to general anesthesia for overall patient satisfaction and reduced morbidity. Short term pain control is definitely improved with spinal anesthesia and new and improved methods for providing longer term analgesia may make this anesthetic technique even more beneficial, especially if contemplating same day discharge and reduced hospital stay.

Author details

W. Scott Jellish* and Steven Edelstein

*Address all correspondence to: wjellis@lumc.edu

Department of Anesthesiology, Loyola University Medical Center, Maywood, USA

References

[1] Mixter WJ, Barr JS. Rupture of the intervertebral disk with involvement of the spinal cord. NEJM 1934;211:210-15.

[2] Williams RW. Microlumbar discectomy: A conservative surgical approach to a virgin herniated lumbar spine. Spine 1978;3:175-82.

[3] Jellish WS, Thalji Z, Stevenson K, et al. A prospective randomized study comparing short and intermediate term perioperative outcomes after spinal or general anesthesia for lumbar disk and laminectomy surgery. Anesth Analg 1996; 83: 559-64.

[4] Bridenbaugh PO, Greene NM. Spinal (subarachnoid) neural blockade. In: Cousin MJ, Bridenbsaugh PO. (ed.) Clinical anesthesia and pain management 3rd Ed. Philadelphia: 1998 p202-241.

[5] Silver DJ, Dunsmore Rh, Dickson Cm. Spinal anesthesia for lumbar disc surgery. Anesth Analg 1976; 550-54.

[6] Tetzloff JE, O'Hara J, Bell G, et al. Influence of baricity on the outcome of spinal anesthesia with bupivacaine for lumbar spine surgery. Reg Anesth 1995;20: 533-37.

[7] Gissen AJ, Covino BG, Gregus J. Differential sensitivities of mammalian nerve fibers to local anesthetic agents. Anesthesiology 1980;53:467-74.

[8] Rung GW, Williams D, Gelb DE, et al. Isobaric spinal anesthesia for lumbar disk surgery. Anesth Analg 1997;84:1165-166.

[9] Laasko E, Pitkanen M, Kytta J, Rosenberg DN. Knee chest vs horizontal side position during induction of spinal anesthesia in patients undergoing lumbar disc surgery. Br J Anaesth 1997;79:609-11.

[10] Reina MA, de Leon-Cassola OA, Lopez A, et al. An scanning electron microscopy in vitro study of dural lesions produced by 25-gauge Quincke and Whitacre needles evaluated by electron microscopy. Reg Anesth Pain Med 2000;25:393-402.

[11] Hebl JR, Horlocker TT, Kopp SL, et al. Neuraxial blockade in patients with preexisting spinal stenosis, lumbar disk disease, or prior spine surgery: Efficacy and neurologic complications. Anesth Analg 2010;111:1511-19.

[12] Goddard M, Smith PD. Spinal anaesthesia for spinal surgery. Anaesth 2006;61:723-24.

[13] Schneider M, Ettlin T, Kaurfmann M, et al. Transient neurologic toxicity after hyperbaric subarachnoid anesthesia with 5% lidocaine. Anesth Analg 1993;76:1154-71.

[14] Zaric D, Christiansen C, Pace NL, et al. Transient neurologic symptoms (TNS) following spinal anaesthesia with lidocaine versus other local anaesthetics. Cochrane Database Syst Rev 4 D003006 2005.

[15] Greene NM. Distribution of local anesthetics in the subarachnoid space. Anesth Analg 1985;64:715-30.

[16] Shesky MC, Rocco AG, Bizzarri-Schmidt M, et al. A Dose-response study of bupivacaine for spinal anesthesia. Anesth Analg 1983;63:931-5.

[17] Bouaziz H, Tong C, Eisenach JC. Postoperative analgesia from intrathecal neostigmine in sheep. Anesth Analg 1995; 80:1140-44.

[18] Brown DL. Spinal, epidural, and caudal anesthesia. In: Churchill Livingstone Elsevier Miller's Anesthesia 7th Ed. Philadelphia: 2010: 1611-1637.

[19] Kuraishi Y, Hirota N, Sato Y, et al. Noradrenergic inhibition and the release of substance P from the primary afferents in the rabbit spinal dorsal horn. Brain Res 1985;359: 177–82.

[20] Jellish WS, Abodeely A, Fluder EM, Shea J. The effect of spinal bupivacaine in combination with either epidural clonidine and/or 0.5% bupivacaine administered at the incision site on postoperative outcome in patients undergoing lumbar laminectomy. Anesth Analg 2003;96:874-80.

[21] Farmery AD, Wilson-MacDonald J. The Analgesic effect of epidural clonidine after spinal surgery: A randomized placebo-controlled trial. Anesth Analg 2009;108:631-4.

[22] Kakiuchi M. Reduction of blood loss during spinal surgery by epidural blockade under normotensive general anesthesia. Spine 1997;22:89-94.

[23] Cousins MJ, Bromage PR. Epidural neural blockage. In: Cousins MJ, Bridenbaugh PO (ed). Clinical Anesthesia and Management of Pain. Phildelphia: 1988 p 253-360.

[24] Goddard M, Smith PD. Spinal anaesthesia for spinal surgery. Anaesth 2006;61:723-24.

[25] McClain RF, Kalfus I, Bell GR, et al. Comparison of spinal and general anesthesia in lumbar laminectomy surgery: A case controlled analysis of 400 patients. J Neurosurg Spine 2005;2:17-22.

[26] Tetzloff JE, Dilger JA, Kodsy M et al. Spinal anesthesia for elective spine surgery. J Clin Anesthesia 1998;10:666-69.

[27] Attari MA, Mirhosseini SA, Honarmad A, et al. Spinal anesthesia versus general anesthesia for elective lumbar spine surgery: A randomized clinical trial. J Res Med Sci 2011;16:524-29.

[28] Kara I, Celik JB, Bahar OC, et al. Comparison of spinal and general anesthesia in lumbar disc surgery. J Neuro Sci (Turkish) 2011;28:487-96.

[29] Sadrolsadat SH, Mahdavi AR, Moharari RS, et cl. A Prospective randomized trial comparing the technique of spinal and general anesthesia for lumbar disk surgery: A study of 100 cases. Surgical Neurology 2009;71:60-5.

[30] Tetzloff JE, O'Hara JF, Yoon JH, et al. Heart rate variability and the prone position under general vs spinal anesthesia. J Clin Anesth 1998;10:656-9.

[31] Hackel DB, Sancetta SM, Kleinerman J. Effect of hypotension due to spinal anesthesia on coronary blood flow and myocardial metabolism in man. Circulation 1956;13:92-7.

[32] Covino BG. Rationale for spinal anesthesia. Int Anesthesiol Clinics 1989;27:8-12.

[33] Eisenach J, Detweiler D, Hood D. Hemodynamics and analgesic actions of epidurally administered clonidine. Anesthesiology 1993;78:277-87.

[34] Lund C. Quitzau S, Greulich A, et al. Comparison of the effects of extradural clonidine with those of morphine on postoperative pain, stress response cardiopulmonary function and motor and sensory block. Br J Anaesth 1989;643:516-9.

[35] Bonhomme V, Doll A, Dewandre PY, et al. Epidural administration of low dose morphine combined with clonidine for postoperative analgesia after lumbar disc surgery. J Neurosurg Anesth 2002;14:1-6.

[36] Cherian MN, Matthews MP, Chandry MJ. Local wound Infiltration with bupivacaine in lumbar laminectomy. Surg Neurol 1997;47:120-5.

[37] Gorfine SR, Onel E, Patou G, Krivokapic. Bupivacaine extended release liposome injection for prolonged postsurgical analgesia in patients undergoing horrhoidectomy: A multicenter randomized, double blind, placebo controlled trial. Dis Colon Rectum 2011;54 1552-9.

[38] Sun Ko. Spinal anaesthesia following previous spinal surgery. European J Anaesth 1994;11: 321-33.

[39] McDaniel MD, Pearce WH, Yao JS, et al. Sequential changes in coagulation and platelet function following femorotibial bypass. J Vasc Surg 1984;26:1-8.

[40] Rosenfeld BA, Beattie C, Christopherson R, et al. The effects of different anesthetic regimens on fibrinolysis and the development of post-operative arterial thrombosis. Anesthesiology 1993;79:435-43.

[41] Dripps RD, Vandam LD. Long term follow-up of patients who received10,098 spinal anesthetics. I. Failure to discover major neurological sequelae. JAMA 1954; 156:1486-91.

[42] Upton AR, McComas AJ. The double crush in nerve entrapment syndromes. Lancet 1973;302:359-62.

[43] Rigler M, Drasner K, Krejcie TC, et al. Cauda equina syndrome after continuous spinal anesthesia. Anesth Analg 1991;72;275-81.

[44] Pollard JB. Cardiac arrest during spinal anesthesia: Common mechanisms and strategies for prevention. Anesth Analg 2001;92:252-6.

[45] Sancetta SM, Lynn B, Simeone FA, et al. Studies of hemodynamic changes in humans following induction of low and high spinal anesthesia: I. General considerations of the problem. The changes in cardiac output, brachial arterial pressure, peripheral and pulmonary oxygen contents and peripheral blood flows induced by spinal anesthesia in humans not undergoing surgery. Circulation 1952;6:559-71.

[46] Mackey DC, Carpenter RL, Thompson GE, et al. Bradycardia and asystole during spinal anesthesia: A report of three cases without morbidity. Anesthesiology 1989;70:866-8.

[47] Campagna JA, Carter R. Clinical relevance of the Bezold-Jarisch reflex. Anesthesiology 2003;98:1250-60.

[48] Kinsella SM, Tuckey JP. Perioperative bradycardia and asytole: A relationship to vasovagal syncope and the Bezold-Jarisch reflex. Br J Anaesth 2001;86:859-69.

[49] Young DV. Comparison of Local, Spinal and general anaesthesia for inguinal herniorrhaphy. Am J Surg 1987;153:560-3.

[50] Uribe JE, Koller J. Omar H, et al. Brachial plexus injury following spine surgery. J Neurolog Spine 2010;13:552-8.

[51] Bekar A, Tureyen K, Aksoy K. Unilateral blindness due to patient positioning during cervical syringomyelia surgery, unilateral blindness after prone positioning. Neurosurg Anesth 1996;8:227-9.

[52] Grossman W, Ward WT. Central retinal artery occlusion after scoliosis surgery with a horse shoe headrest: Case report and literature review. Spine 1993;18:1226-28.

[53] Dharmavarm S, Jellish WS, Nockels RS. Effect of prone positioning on hemodynamic and cardiac function during lumbar spine surgery. The Spine Journal 2006;31:1388-93.

Chapter 3

Spinal Anaesthesia for Ambulatory and Short-Stay Plastic Surgery Procedures

Víctor M. Whizar-Lugo, Juan C. Flores-Carrillo, Susana Preciado-Ramírez, Jaime Campos-León and Víctor Silva

Additional information is available at the end of the chapter

http://dx.doi.org/10.5772/58407

1. Introduction

Outpatient and short-stay plastic surgery procedures have increased recently up to 457% [1] due to lower prices, global availability of plastic surgeons, better and safer anaesthetic techniques. This exponential growth has been increased by greater information in the media, most notably by means of the enlightenment shown in the internet. Every day more complex patients force anaesthesiologists to develop better techniques using multimodal approaches before, during and after anaesthesia. Nowadays it is possible to perform ambulatory plastic surgery procedures in people with medical conditions that in the past were rejected; myocardial ischemia, arrhythmias, hypertension, coagulation disorders, lung diseases, diabetes, etcetera. Improved safety and efficacy in all anaesthesia procedures for plastic surgery is mandatory; surgeons, patients, relatives and media have their own concerns regarding anaesthesia patient safety.

Local anaesthesia, plexus nerve blocks and neuroaxial techniques have been reported with excellent results, as well as patient comfort and acceptance. Spinal, epidural or combined spinal-epidural procedures are quite safe and have attained widespread use for patients undergoing ambulatory surgery below the Th3-Th4 spinal level. Spinal anaesthesia for outpatient and short-stay plastic surgery cases have been well accepted by surgeons and patients due to its rapid onset and offset, easy administration, minimal expenses, and almost no side effects or complications. Ambulatory procedures as liposuction, buttocks implants and calf implants, and many more are done properly under spinal anaesthesia. Longer surgeries like abdominoplasty, lower body lift, or combined surgeries involving upper and lower body segments are also done safely under subarachnoid or epidural anaesthesia.[2,3,4] Small gauge pencil point needles have acceptable rates of 0 to 3 % of postdural puncture headache (PDPH);

the most fearful side effect of spinal anaesthesia. There are several choices of local anaesthetics (LAs) available for spinal anaesthesia for ambulatory and short-stay patients, including ropivacaine, levobupivacaine, racemic bupivacaine, prilocaine, mepivacaine, articaine, procaine and chloroprocaine. Although controversial, lidocaine is no longer recommended to be used for spinal anaesthesia. Intraspinal adjuvant drugs like clonidine, dexmedetomidine, morphine, sufentanyl and fentanyl enhance quality and duration of spinal blocks.

Deep venous thrombosis and pulmonary embolism remains the greatest cause of morbidity and mortality in plastic surgery.[5,6,7] Spinal anaesthesia decreases these complications as it facilitates early ambulation. Postoperative pain can be managed with preoperative preemptive analgesia techniques, plus adjuvant drugs injected into the spinal space.

For the purposes of this review we define outpatient surgery cases as those who are discharged the same day of the procedure, and short-stay patients those who remain in the surgical unit or hospital for 24 hours after surgery. This chapter reviews the indications, contraindications, advantages, disadvantages and drugs used for spinal anaesthesia in ambulatory and short-stay plastic surgery procedures.

2. Subarachnoid anaesthesia techniques

There are three ways to perform spinal anaesthesia; single injection, combined spinal-epidural, and continuous subarachnoid anaesthesia with small gauge spinal catheters.

Single injection. Is the most widely used since it is easy to perform, safe, predictable, has low incidence of side effects, and low cost. The addition of adjuvants drugs to LAs provides sufficient time for more prolonged plastic surgical procedures, and therefore is the ideal technique in these patients.[3]

Combined spinal/epidural. Combines the benefits of epidural and subarachnoid anaesthesia, lessening some of the disadvantages of both procedures. This technique allow us to titrate the upper sensory level, to reduce total dose of epidural LAs, and to continue anaesthesia as long as needed.[8,9] It is recommend for long plastic surgeries involving chest, abdomen and extremities in the same patient. Sometimes it is difficult to keep the epidural catheter in place, and it can also migrate outside the epidural space.[10,11]

Continuous spinal anaesthesia. Described by Dean in 1907 [12] was reintroduced by Lemmon in 1940 [13]. The technique had several modifications until Hurley and Lambert [14] introduced the use of thin spinal microcatheters 32-gauge. Nowadays this procedure is underutilized due to several cases of cauda equina syndrome and the FDA recommendation to withdraw the technique. The main advantages of continuous spinal anaesthesia is to allow redosing of small amount of LA to prolong duration of anaesthesia/analgesia and provide better hemodynamic stability.[15] In the field of plastic surgery outpatient and short-stay cases it may be limited for older patients with prolonged procedures below Th8 dermatomes.

Spinal anesthesia is done following anatomical landmarks. The introduction of ultrasound in regional anesthesia is an advanced technique that is now used in difficult cases where anatomy cannot be identified properly, or when a difficult block is anticipated as in morbidly obese or patients with severe anatomic alterations.

3. Indications of spinal anaesthesia

There are two groups of patients who desire plastic surgery procedures: a) Those who undergo surgery for purely aesthetic reasons to look better and b) Those who do it for work, social or professional demands. These are patients with special wishes and needs that most of the times border on perfection, therefore they have poor tolerability for errors or side effects. Complications from anaesthesia are not tolerable, even small or insignificant side effects are not accepted. These patient characteristics demand a careful anaesthesiologist, a cautious anaesthetic plan with some management alternatives ready to be use in order to stay away from mistakes and complications.

Typically spinal anaesthesia is used for surgical procedures below dermatome Th10, involving the abdomen, pelvis, perineum, and lower extremities. Outpatient and short-stay plastic surgery procedures localized up to dermatome Th3-Th4 can be safely done under lumbar spinal anaesthesia, tilting the surgery table in Trendelemburg or reverse Trendelemburg position until the desired surgical level is reached. For example, you can use lumbar subarachnoid block for breast surgery and chest/back liposuction, or abdominoplasty combined with breast surgery.[16,17]

Tables 1 and 2 show our recommendations for outpatient and short-stay cosmetic surgery procedures that can be done under spinal anaesthesia, including surgeries up to Th3-Th4 dermatomes. In some circumstances it is convenient to use combined epidural-intrathecal anaesthesia to ensure sufficient anaesthetic duration, as discussed previously.

Surgery	Spinal		Epidural		Spinal-epidural	
	Anaesthetic	Adjuvant	Anaesthetic	Adjuvant	Anaesthetic	Adjuvant
Liposuction	L, PPX	C, F	L, PPX	C, F	L, PPX	C, F, S
Liposculpture	L, PPX	C, F	L, PPX	C, F	L, PPX	C, F, S
Buttock Implants/fat grafting	L,PPX	C	L, PPX	C	L, PPX	C, F, S
Calf Implants	L, PPX	C	L, PPX	C	L, PPX	C, F, S
Breast and liposuction	PPX	C, F	L, PPX	C, F	L, PPX	C, F. S
Breast only	Not recomended	Not recomended	L, PPX	Not recomended	Not recomended	Not recomended
Perineal procedures	L, PPX	C, F	L, PPX	C, F	Not recomended	Not recomended

L=lidocaine, PPX=Racemic bupivacaine, Levobupivacaine, Ropivacaine, or Mepivacaine

C=Clonidine, F=Fentanyl

Table 1. Ambulatory plastic surgery procedures and neuroaxial anaesthesia.[3]

Surgery	Spinal		Epidural		Spinal-epidural	
	Anaesthetic	Adjuvant	Anaesthetic	Adjuvant	Anaesthetic	Adjuvant
Abdominoplasty (Simple, extended or circular)	PPX	C, F, S, or M	PPX	C, F. M	PPX	C, F, S, or M
Abdominoplasty with breast surgery	PPX	C, F, S, or M	PPX	C, F, M	PPX	C, F, S, or M
Lower body lift	PPX	C, F, S, or M	PPX	C, F, M	PPX	C, F, S, or M
Breast pexia	Not recommended	Not recommended	L, PPX	C, F	Not recommended	Not recommended

L=lidocaine, PPX=Racemic bupivacaine, Levobupivacaine, Ropivacaine, or Mepivacaine,

C=Clonidine, F=Fentanyl. S=Sufentanyl. M=Morphine

Table 2. Short-stay plastic surgery procedures and neuroaxial anaesthesia.[3]

4. Contraindications for spinal anaesthesia

Contraindications are divided into absolute and relative, as shown in table 3. Contraindications for spinal anaesthesia have been changed over time due to advanced equipment such small gauge pencil point spinal needles, small gauge Quincke type spinal needles, special tip designs spinal needles, recent LAs and adjuvants drugs. Patients who wish to fly few days after their surgery should not receive spinal anaesthesia because of the pressure changes in aircraft cabins may facilitate cerebrospinal fluid (CSF) leak through the duramater hole. In addition to these general contraindications, there are few situations where it is not advisable to use spinal anaesthesia in these patients. For example; patients who live far away from where they are operated and are not able or willing to return to this facility, should not receive spinal anaesthesia because the small risk of PDPH. This situation implies that they have to be treated by colleagues at their city of origin and could facilitate unnecessary medical legal problems. With plastic surgeons that require longer surgical times it is better to avoid spinal anaesthesia or advice the patients that they may need general anaesthesia near the end of the procedure.

Absolute

- Patient rejection
- Severe coagulation disorders
- Infection at cutaneous injection site
- Hypovolemia or hemodynamic inestability
- Increased intracranial pressure

Relative

http://dx.doi.org/10.5772/58407

- Sepsis
- Preexisting diseases of the central nervous system
  - Multiple sclerosis
  - Spina bifida
  - Cancer
  - Hydrocephalus derived
- Anticoagulation
- Thrombocytopenia and thrombasthenia
- Severe anatomical deformities
- Preload dependent conditions
  - Aortic stenosis
  - Obstructive hyperthrophic cardiomiopathy
- Air travel in the immediate post anaesthetic period

Table 3. Spinal anaesthesia contraindications

5. Advantages and complications of spinal anaesthesia

Subarachnoid anaesthesia is an easy procedure that provides a deep and fast surgical block through the injection of small dose of LA into the lumbar spinal space.[18,19] Even though lumbar volume of CSF is the main determinant of the effects produced by intrathecal injection of LA solutions, duration and spread of spinal anaesthesia can be easily manipulated with type/dose of LAs, baricity of the solution, as well as the addition of preservative free adjuvant drugs like opioids and/or alpha$_2$-adrenergic agonists.[19,20] Although some aspects of this technique are controversial, nowadays it is known to be safer than epidural anaesthesia,[21] with many advantages over other anaesthetic procedures, fewer side effects and uncommon severe complications.

Advantages. Subarachnoid anaesthesia for ambulatory and short-stay plastic surgery patients is characterized by rapid onset and convenient offset, quick and simple administration, inexpensive, with minimal side effects and very few complications. It offers many advantages for this type of patients as it can be used for procedures below Th3-Th4 such as breast surgery, abdominal procedures, liposuction and many more surgeries (Tables 1 and 2). The use of small gauge pencil point spinal needles has reduced to 0-3% the incidence of PDPH, even in young and outpatients. Spinal anaesthesia is more predictable and safer than epidural or general anaesthesia. The likelihood of neural damage is reduced when compared to peripheral nerve blocks. Regional anaesthesia procedures, including subarachnoid anaesthesia, have better pain control, attenuation of the surgical stress response, preserve perioperative immune function, better preservation of oxygenation and pulmonary residual functional capacity, improved visceral vascular flow, early recovery of postoperative ileum, and reduced venous thrombotic disease and pulmonary embolism.

Complications and disadvantages. Bradycardia and hypotension are the most frequent cardiovascular side effects associated with spinal anaesthesia and are related to the secondary sympathetic block. Total dose/volume of injected LAs have a direct relationship with the cardiovascular response. Bradycardia and arterial hypotension are easy to treat with intravenous fluids and vasoactive drugs. Sudden cardiac arrest is observed with an estimated incidence of 0.7 to 0.15%.[22,23,24,25] Changing patient position and hypovolemia are factors related to sudden cardiac arrest, this situation can take place during extensive liposuction or abdominoplasty-liposuction. In these patients it is very important to use preventive treatment as well as to establish proper therapy immediately.

Nerve damage is the most feared side effect of spinal anaesthesia. It can be secondary to local neurotoxicity of LAs or adjuvant drugs, direct needle damage, haematoma or spinal infection. Cauda equina syndrome and transitory neurological symptoms (TNS) due to posterior nerve roots irritation at their entry to the spinal cord [26] are the most neurological controversial side effects. Several mechanisms have been proposed to explain them. Local neurotoxicity after spinal injection of any LA is an issue of concern raised after the first published data by Schneider.[27] Follow up of patients who received uncomplicated spinal anaesthesia had shown that some developed pain in the buttocks and/or lower extremities after an initial full recovery from spinal anaesthesia. This painful condition that occurs in the immediate post-operative period is known as TNS, and last up to 5 days. Numerous articles have been published showing that subarachnoid LAs are not free of neurotoxicity; all of them are neurotoxic when injected inside the spinal space, having a different grade of toxicity. [27,28,29,30] Takenami et al [26] found in rats that supraclinical concentration of lidocaine initially is limited to the posterior roots at their entry to the spinal cord. Zong et al found that spinal ropivacaine 0.75-1.0% induced neurotoxicity after repeated injections in rats; infiltration of inflammatory cells, vacuolation of myelin sheaths and axons, abnormal morphology of neurons and apoptosis in the spinal cord, mainly in posterior roots and the adjacent posterior white matter.[31]

In summary, spinal lidocaine is the most neurotoxic LA, followed in descending order of toxicity by bupivacaine, levobupivacaine, ropivacaine, articaine, chloroprocaine and procaine.

Postdural puncture headache. This complication is no longer a major concern with a rate of 0 to 3% when pencil point G-27 to G-25, Quincke point G-27,or special tip like Atraucan spinal needles are used. Even in younger outpatients who were considered at high risk for developing PDPH, this side effect is seldom observed.[32,33] Post dural puncture headache is attributed to CSF leak to the extradural space through the hole in the dura. Reina et al [34] found that G-25 Quincke needles produced well defined dural holes without inflammatory reaction, while the G-25 Whitacre needles leave a dural hole with separation and disruption of the collagen fibers and a inflammatory component. They argue that the edema that occurs by this inflammatory reaction is responsible for the closure of the dural hole, which clinically lowers the incidence of PDPH by preventing further loss of CSF. Post dural puncture headache can prolong the convalescence of patients and be a determining factor for hospital readmission. Seventy to 90% of patients have a spontaneous resolution in one to six weeks after dural puncture. Conservative management involves bed rest, fluids, analgesics and caffeine.

Epidural blood patch is seldom needed for PDPH after subarachnoid anaesthesia done with pencil point needles.

Failed spinal. There are several factors to explain this malfunction; partial position of spinal needle tip into the subdural or epidural space, inadequate dose, expired LAs, injection into a dural sac appendix (Tarlov's cyst), low spinal tap, inadequate accumulation of hyperbaric LA in sacral roots, and on occasions when surgery is prolonged beyond the time of the spinal anaesthesia.[35] When a subarachnoid block fails, 20-30 minutes must elapse before it is repeated so as to avoid the possibility of additive effects over the first dose of LA. It is important to be sure that the first injected LA has reached its maximum effect, if any. Remember that the spread of LAs may be very slow in some patients, therefore a waiting time of 20 to 30 minutes ensures that most of the LA which access the subarachnoid space is fixed in the neural tissue. The second injection done at the same space, or even better in upper spaces, usually produces a proper subarachnoid block. It has been recommended not to use opioids during the second attempt (if opioids were used in the first attempt) to avoid eventually delayed respiratory depression. It is also wise not to use vasoconstrictors in the second injection that could lead to severe nerve damage by ischemia.[36,37] The addition of clonidine might be safe during the second spinal block as intratecal doses of this drug are very wide (30 to 450 μg).

Arachnoiditis. Recent studies on the incidence of arachnoiditis secondary to neuroaxial anaesthesia seems to point out this new entity as a ghost, as a deleterious effect that we must consider each time that a patient will undergo a neuroaxial injection. This entity may present initially as TNS, cauda equina syndrome or conus medullaris, and then evolve radiculitis, fibrosis, scarring of the dural sac, deformities, pachymeningitis, syringomyelia, and pseudo-meningocele among others. It has been associated with neuroaxial anaesthesia after traumatic punctures, LAs, detergents, antiseptics, preservatives and other substances injected by accident or intentionally into the subarachnoid, subdural or peridural space.[38]

Total spinal block. It can happen during extradural block attempt with inadverted dural puncture and the injection of high volume of LAs. During spinal anaesthesia LAs seldom reach an unwanted high metameric level. This situation happens with inappropriate high doses of LAs, neglect manipulation of patient position when injected with hypo or hyperbaric LAs. If the level is too high, it may be accompanied by bradycardia, cardiac arrest and or respiratory failure requiring pharmacologic and ventilatory support.

Bleeding. The development of cerebral or spinal haematomas subsequent to spinal anaesthesia is a serious and rare complication which mandates prompt diagnosis, and immediate surgery. A closed claims study in Finland during 2000/2009 [22] found an incidence of neuroaxial haematoma after spinal anaesthesia of 1:775,000, which is lesser than epidural anaesthesia 1:26,400 and combined epidural-spinal 1:17,800. Castillo et al. in Catalonia Spain [39] reported an approximated incidence of one haematoma per 150,000 neuroaxial anaesthesias (0.6 per 100,000 spinal anaesthesias versus 0.7 per 100,000 epidural anaesthesias). When performing neuroaxial anaesthesia it is important to adhere to ASRA guidelines [40] avoiding regional anaesthesia in patients at risk of bleeding such as coagulation abnormalities, anticoagulation therapy. Remember that certain conditions like advanced age, anomalies of the vertebral column or spinal cord, and difficult neuroaxial blocks can increase the risk of bleeding.

Trauma and infection. There have been reports of nerve damage by direct trauma produced by the spinal needle, and also there are reports of infections manifested as meningitis or epidural abscesses after neuroaxial anaesthesia. Instances of either occurrence are exceedingly uncommon.[25]

As reviewed in the previous paragraphs, severe complications secondary to spinal anaesthesia are extremely rare and therefore difficult to study. Auroy et al [25] in their prospective study conducted in France with 756 anaesthesiologists found that the incidence of deleterious events after regional anaesthesia were rare; they found only 98 incidents in 103,730 cases. There were 40,640 cases of spinal anaesthesia with cardiac arrest in 26 of whom 6 died, (6.4 ± 1.2./ 10,000 patients) which was significant ($p < 0.05$) when compare with other regional anaesthesia techniques. There were 21 neurological complications (radiculopathy, cauda equina syndrome, paraplegia). Two thirds of the patients with neurologic deficits had either a paresthesia during needle placement or pain on injection and 75 % of the neurologic deficits after non-traumatic spinal anaesthesia occurred in patients who had received 5% hyperbaric lidocaine.

6. Drugs for spinal anaesthesia

There are two groups of drugs used for spinal anaesthesia; LAs and adjuvant drugs. The latter are used to enhance the performance of spinal anaesthesia and or to lower doses of LAs and their corresponding side effects. They can be injected through a spinal needle or multiple doses through a spinal catheter.

Systemic toxicity of LAs is not an issue in subarachnoid anaesthesia, since the dosages used are very small compared with the epidural doses. However, due to the increasing use of combined neuroaxial anaesthesia (subarachnoid-epidural) and injections of higher doses of lidocaine during liposuction, abdominoplasty or neck and face lift, it is important to bear in mind the possibility of systemic toxicity manifested by seizures, coma, arrhythmias, or heart failure.

The choice of the spinal LA is determined taking into account the type and duration of plastic surgery procedures, patient health condition, facilities where the operation is performed, the experience of the anaesthesiologist, dexterity of surgeons, and availability of drugs. Also, it is important where the patient lives, or if he/she are tourist patients from a remote place.

The anaesthetic profile of each intrathecal drug is the most important parameter that should be considered when planning subarachnoid anaesthesia.

Local anaesthetics. Due to the unresolved dispute over local neurotoxicity of intrathecal lidocaine,[41] some researchers have attempted to determine the usefulness of other LAs in the field of ambulatory and short-stay surgery, keeping in mind that recovery time after spinal anaesthesia is important for patients, physicians, third party payers and surgical units. There are quite a few choices of LAs for outpatient and short-stay spinal anaesthesia; bupivacaine, levobupivacaine, ropivacaine, mepivacaine, prilocaine, chloroprocaine, procaine, articaine, and lidocaine.[3,42,43]

http://dx.doi.org/10.5772/58407

Local anaesthetics		Adjuvants
Amino-ester	**Amino-amide**	
Procaine	Lidocaine	Fentanyl
2-cloroprocaine	Articaine	Sufentanyl
Tetracaine	Bupivacaine	Morphine
	Levobupivacaine	Clonidine
	Ropivacaine	Dexmedetomidine
	Mepivacaine	
	Prilocaine	
	Etidocaine	

Table 4. Drugs for spinal anaesthesia for ambulatory and short-stay plastic surgery procedures

The amino-amide pipecoloxylidides (PPX) family of LAs incorporate four drugs: racemic bupivacaine, mepivacaine, ropivacaine and levobupivacaine. All of them are used in spinal anaesthesia for ambulatory cases, in particular bupivacaine. Changes in the total dose and/or adding some adjuvant drugs has been a growing field in this line of research/clinical practice. Ropivacaine and levobupivacaine have not been approved all over the world for intrathecal use, however, multiple reports and the fact that they are made preservatives free make them safe when injected inside the spinal space.[43,44,45]

In the following paragraphs we briefly review some LAs used in spinal anaesthesia for outpatient and short-stay cases in various surgical procedures, and analyze their results to use them in ambulatory and brief-stay plastic surgery patients. We describe the amide class of LAs first, followed by the ester type.

Lidocaine. Is the most studied/used LA. During the last two decades there has been an increase in the number of patients implicating lidocaine as a possible source of neurotoxicity resulting in temporary and permanent neurologic damage after subarachnoid anaesthesia. Nowadays cauda equina is seldom reported after spinal lidocaine, but TNS are the most reported deleterious side effects. The risk to develop TNS is significantly higher after spinal lidocaine compared to spinal bupivacaine, prilocaine, procaine, levobupivacaine, ropivacaine, and chloroprocaine (7.31 (95% confidence interval (CI) 4.16 to 12.86).[46] Fortunately, TNS symptoms last no more than five days, without permanent neural damage. Among other causes, early ambulation is one of the factors that has been associated with the development of toxicity symptoms, so in ambulatory and short-stay patients spinal lidocaine could be contraindicated.

Although spinal lidocaine use is controversial, some authors still use it for short procedures. A dose of 40 mg is sufficient and compared with 7.5 mg of bupivacaine.[19] A dose of 15 mg of lidocaine plus 15 μg of sufentanyl produces excellent anaesthesia and recovery time better than 50 mg of lidocaine alone, however 50% develops pruritus.[47] Frey et al compared in healthy volunteers [48] 100 mg of lidocaine, bupivacaine 15 mg and 15 mg of tetracaine-the three hyperbaric-and found that lidocaine has the best recovery profile, although there were patient dependent variables between the three studied LAs, with some subjects recovering quickly among those treated with bupivacaine or tetracaine. No major differences were found between 80 mg of either spinal isobaric lidocaine 2% or spinal isobaric mepivacaine 2% for ambulatory arthroscopic surgery. Neither group had TNS.[49] Prilocaine, mepivacaine, articaine, bupivacaine, ropivacaine, and procaine at low doses have been suggested as alternatives to spinal lidocaine.

Articaine. A 4-methyl-3(2-[propylamino] propionamido)-2-thiophenecarboxylic acid, methyl ester hydrochloride, originally named carticaine was first prepared by Rusching *et al* in 1969. Introduced in dentistry in 1973, it entered clinical practice in Germany in 1976 under the changed name of articaine. It is the only amide LA that contains a thiophene ring and an additional ester ring. Recent investigations have demonstrated its usefulness in spinal anaesthesia for ambulatory short cases. In addition to its fast onset and short duration of motor blockade, it has low local neurotoxicity.[50,51,52] Doses from 50 to 80 mg of 2% or 3% plain or hyperbaric articaine produces satisfactory anaesthesia for about 1 hour, with full recovery in 3.5 hours. Hyperbaric articaine was compared with hyperbaric bupivacaine in similar surgeries, and the results have shown a quicker onset of sensory and sympathetic block in the articaine group than in the bupivacaine group, but hypotension was more frequent and faster with articaine.[53] Hendriks et al [54] compared 50 mg of plain articaine versus 50 mg of plain prilocaine in day-case knee arthroscopy patients and found that full motor function recovery was shorter after articaine than prilocaine [mean (SD) 140 [33] versus 184 [46] min, respectively, $p<0.001$]. Time to spontaneous voiding was shorter after articaine than prilocaine [mean (SD) 184 [39] versus 227 [45] min, respectively, $p<0.001$]. One patient in the articaine group reported mild TNS limited to the first postoperative day, but there were no significant differences in adverse effects between the groups.[50] Addition of fentanyl 10 μg improved analgesia and reduced postoperative analgesic consumption without prolonging motor block nor delaying total recovery.[55,56]

Bupivacaine. Is an old drug that has stood the test of time. It is a racemic LA containing two stereoisomers, $S^-$and R^+, the latter being the most toxic. Since the controversy of spinal lidocaine neurotoxicity, bupivacaine is probably the more used LA in subarachnoid anaesthesia. Its intrathecal potency is similar to levobupivacaine and stronger than ropivacaine: ratios are 0.97 (95% CI: 0.81-1.17) for levobupivacaine/bupivacaine, 0.65 (95% CI: 0.54-0.80) for ropivacaine/ bupivacaine, and 0.68 (95% CI: 0.55-0.84) for ropivacaine/levobupivacaine.[57] Although it is an adequate substitute for intrathecal lidocaine for outpatient and short-stay surgery, the usual doses of 15 to18 mg may be reduced 8 to 10 mg to prevent urinary retention and delayed home discharge. In addition, almost no possibility of TNS favors the use of bupivacaine for ambulatory plastic surgery. A systematic review by Nair et al [58] suggested that 4-5 mg of hyperbaric bupivacaine can effectively produce spinal anaesthesia for knee arthroscopy with unilateral positioning. Casati et al [59] compared 8 mg 0.5 % hyperbaric bupivacaine versus sciatic-femoral nerve block with mepivacaine and found that to carry out peripheral nerve blocks require more time than to perform spinal anaesthesia. Patients under spinal anaesthesia had shorter time block, but took longer to urinate without affecting discharge time. A small dose of 4 mg hyperbaric bupivacaine 0.25% reduces the height of sensory block and motor block duration. Doses of 3 and 4 mg of spinal hyperbaric 0.5% bupivacaine, with fentanyl 25 μg, or without the opioid can be used safely in lower extremity surgery and can provide rapid and safe release criteria.[60] Intrathecal injection of 9.7 mg of isobaric bupivacaine acts five minutes faster than hyperbaric bupivacaine, although at 15 min level of sensory and motor block have similar characteristics of hyperbaric bupivacaine.[61] For ambulatory cosmetic short procedures doses of 8 to 10 mg hyperbaric 0.5%-0.75% bupivacaine are adequate, for short-stay procedures like abdominoplasty plus breast surgery doses from 15 up to 22 mg can be used safely, but full recovery time will be affected.

Levobupivacaine. It is the last LA introduced in clinical practice back in 1999. It is an L-stereo-isomer with a longer duration of action, a clinical profile similar to racemic bupivacaine, but with less toxicity. The lethal dose of intravenous levobupivacaine is 1.3 to 1.6 times greater than racemic bupivacaine, and both have equipotent anaesthetic effect via neuroaxial. Some animal's studies have shown no damage or minimal harm to the spinal cord or cauda equina. [62,63] In contrast, Takenami et al found axonal degeneration in rats injected with spinal levobupivacaine.[30] There are numerous clinical studies recommending spinal levobupivacaine in ambulatory surgery. Doses from 7.5 to 15 mg 0.5% hyperbaric/isobaric levobupivacaine produced satisfactory anaesthesia.[64,65] Smaller doses with added adjuvants have been reported for ambulatory cases; in gynecological patients 3 mg along with 10 μg fentanyl may be used safely,[66] 5 or 7.5 mg 0.5% intrathecal levobupivacaine plus fentanyl 25 μg for ambulatory patients undergoing inguinal herniorraphy provides good quality spinal anaesthesia and minimizes the need for intra-operative analgesia.[67] In a double-blinded study Sanansilp et al [68] compared spinal isobaric or hyperbaric 0.42% levobupivacaine. They found that hyperbaric levobupivacaine spread higher than the isobaric form, suggesting that the former is more predictable. In elderly patients spinal levobupivacaine has better hemodynamic stability compared with bupivacaine.[69]

Although intrathecal levobupivacaine is safe, there have been reported cases of cauda equina syndrome and TNS. Twenty mg of isobaric levobupivacaine produce less TNS than 80 mg of isobaric lidocaine (0.33% versus 26.6%, p=0.002).[70] We describe a 38 year old patient who developed TNS 27 hours after abdominoplasty/liposuction done under spinal anaesthesia with 15 mg of 0.65% hyperbaric levobupivacaine and 30 μg clonidine.[71]

Ropivacaine. Identified by Ekenstam in 1957, ropivacaine was introduced in clinical loco regional and epidural anesthesia in 1997. It is the first available L-isomer LA for human use. It is less soluble than bupivacaine, and is the least toxic of the PPX family. The possibility of TNS is 0-1%. Shortly after its introduction, ropivacaine was safely used for spinal anaesthesia in the ambulatory setting. It is one third less potent compared to bupivacaine or levobupivacaine.[43] Hyperbaric 0.5% ropivacaine is superior to 0.5% hyperbaric bupivacaine outpatients, since motor and sensitive block duration are significantly shorter than bupivacaine, with better cardiovascular stability.[72] Like levobupivacaine, low doses of ropivacaine are useful in outpatients; several investigative protocols reports small doses from 5 to 10 mg were sufficient in various types of outpatient surgeries like anorectal,[73] knee arthroscopy,[74] herniorraphy.

[75] Gautier et al [76] found that 12 mg intrathecal ropivacaine are equivalent to 8 mg of bupivacaine, with no additional benefits in outpatients undergoing knee arthroscopies. The accidental injection of 1.0% ropivacaine 30 mg without serious side effects suggests us that higher doses may be used when are needed for procedures in thoracic dermatomes, even for ambulatory patients.[77]

Doses from 4 up to 30 mg of isobaric or hyperbaric 0.75 or 1% ropivacaine can be safely used for ambulatory or short-stay plastic surgery procedures.

Mepivacaine. This LA has been used intrathecally since 1960. It has a short onset with intermediate duration and low toxicity. Its hepatic metabolism is fast and is excreted by the kidneys. Its clinical profile is similar to lidocaine, with a relative potency of 1.3:1. Spinal mepivacaine produces neurological tissue damage with infiltration of macrophages and destruction of the myelin sheaths and axons in rats. The damage was localized in the proximal portion of the posterior nerve roots, the entry zone into the spinal cord, or the fasciculus gracilis of the posterior white mater.[28] Transient neurological symptoms occurs between 0 and 30%. A study of 1273 ambulatory patients managed with mepivacaine 1.5% intrathecal-epidural or intrathecal showed that 1.7% of spinal anaesthesia were inadequate and 6.4% had TNS. The average age of patients who developed TNS was 48 ± 14 years), significantly older than those who had not TNS (41 ± 16) (p <0.001).[78] Pawlowski et al [79] prospectively studied the anaesthetic recovery profile in 60 outpatients managed with 60 and 80 mg intrathecal mepivacaine and concluded that both doses are adequate, although patients who were managed with 60 mg recovered faster (20 to 30 minutes) without any side effects. The same authors found no major differences between lidocaine and mepivacaine spinal anaesthesia; time to ambulation and voiding were longer in patients who received mepivacaine as was time to epidural first dose. Neither group had TNS symptoms. Lidocaine and mepivacaine are both appropriate spinal anaesthetics for ambulatory orthopedic lower extremity procedures.[80] Adding fentanyl 10 μg to 30 mg isobaric spinal mepivacaine 1.5% produces reliable anaesthesia, hastens block regression, shortens recovery, and facilitates earlier ambulation for patients undergoing unilateral knee arthroscopy.[81]

2-Chloroprocaine. It is an ester LA suitable for short procedures under spinal anaesthesia. Preservative free chloroprocaine has been used instead of intrathecal lidocaine in order to avoid TNS. It has an antagonistic effect on k and μ opioid receptors, which may interfere with neuroaxial opioid administration. Spinal 2-chloroprocaine, 10 mg/mL 35, 40, 45, 50 and 60 mg provide consistent sensory and motor block for ambulatory surgery, while reducing the doses to 35 and 40 mg resulted in a spinal block with faster ambulation. Even though 20 mg and 30 mg doses can produce adequate sensory anaesthesia for short surgical procedures, less motor block and some sacral sparing should be anticipated. Most studies recommend doses from 30 to 60 mg. A dose of 10 mg produces brief and inconsistent sensory anaesthesia, it can be considered a no effect dose.[82] Hejtmanek and Pollock [83] review 503 ambulatory patients managed with spinal chloroprocaine (median dose 40 mg, range 20-60 mg) and found that times from injection to ambulation and discharge were 107±24 and 171±45 min, respectively, shorter than spinal lidocaine (155±40 and 224±57 min) (p<0.05), with no reports of TNS.

Compared with 40 mg articaine, 40 mg of chloroprocaine had similar onset and maximal spread, but recovery from motor block was clearly faster with chloroprocaine.[84] Adding fentanyl appears to lengthen the surgical block without prolonging discharge time. Five possible cases of TNS following spinal chloroprocaine in over 4000 patients, and a regressive incomplete cauda equina syndrome have been described.[85] To sum up, the short duration of spinal chloroprocaine makes it a strong contender for outpatient anaesthesia. It appears to have a lower risk of TNS than lidocaine.

Procaine. This amino-ester LA has been used in the subarachnoid space for short surgeries since the beginning of last century. Its onset of action is slower than chloroprocaine, and only lasts 30 to 60 minutes. Although procaine produces local toxicity, it is the least neurotoxic LA when injected inside the spinal space.[28] TNS have an incidence 0 to 6%. Johnson and Swanson [86] reported a patient with permanent cauda equina syndrome after 150 mg of 10% procaine. Hodgson [87] used 100 mg hyperbaric spinal procaine versus 50 mg hyperbaric lidocaine in outpatient arthroscopy and found that the first had a higher rate of anaesthetic failure (17% versus 3%), and higher incidence of nausea (17% versus 3%). TNS incidence was lower with procaine (6% vs. 24%). Procaine has been considered as an acceptable alternative to intrathecal lidocaine in ambulatory patients.

When choosing a LA for subarachnoid anaesthesia it is important to keep in mind that hyperbaric forms have a wider intrathecal diffusion compared to isobaric solutions, and therefore they are useful for higher dermatomes surgical procedures. The isobaric LAs are better for pelvic and lower extremity surgeries. Epinephrine is no longer recommended since it lengthens recovery time. It is always wise to consider that operating time is longer than the surgeon's estimate, as there are many timeouts prolonging the surgery. Furthermore, sometimes the original cosmetic surgical plans are modified during surgery, thereby prolonging the surgical procedure.[3] Tables 5 and 6 shows LAs and adjuvants mixtures according to the expected operating times. Note that this includes surgeries less than an hour long, which is uncommon (review of scars, liposuction of small areas, perineal). For these ultra short cases the combination of procaine+clonidine+fentanyl is excellent, without the ghost of TNS. Low doses of PPX local anaesthetics are good, but usually last longer and in a very busy facility, could prolong discharge. Doses 5 to 8 mg of ropivacaine, bupivacaine or levobupivacaine provide up to 150 minutes of intrathecal anaesthesia. This is sufficient time for most outpatient procedures in cosmetic surgery. Prolongation of the action of the LAs by adding clonidine is dose related; 150 to 300 μg can prolong spinal anaesthesia up to 4-5 hours. Drowsiness, bradycardia and hypotension are more frequent with the higher doses, but easy to treat.

In our Plastic Surgery Center the most used spinal LA for ambulatory and short-stay patients are hyperbaric bupivacaine 0.5% and 0.75%, hyperbaric ropivacaine 0.75%, and hyperbaric levobupivacaine 0.5%. We avoid the use of intrathecal lidocaine. For brief ambulatory cases we prefer to use low dose of any PPX family LA, plus clonidine 30 to 50 μg. If the ambulatory procedure is over two hours it is advisable to use regular doses of LAs, and add clonidine in doses from 75 up to 150 μg. We do not recommend spinal opioids in ambulatory cases given the likelihood of pruritus and urinary retention. For short-stay long procedures we use hyperbaric bupivacaine 15 to 25 mg, hyperbaric ropivacaine 15 to 30 mg, or hyperbaric levobupivacaine 15 up to 25 mg. Most of our short-stay patients also receive spinal clonidine 150 to 300 μg, with or without fentanyl 12.5 to 25 μg, or sufentanyl 10 μg. Morphine (100 to 200 μg) is seldom used, even in short-stay patients.

Surgery	Local anaesthetic concentration and total dose in mg			
	Ropivacaine 0.75%	Levobupivacaine 0.75%	Bupivacaine 0.5 a 0.75%	Lidocaine 2%**
Liposucction with buttocks fat grafting	10 a 22.5	7.5 – 18	7.5 – 15	50 -100
Liposculpture	10 a 22.5	7.5 – 18	7.5 – 15	50 - 100
Buttocks implants	15	10	10	100
Calf implants	15	10	10	100
Breast implants combined with body liposuction°	22.5	18	18	No

* Hyperbaric local anaesthetics. The addition of adjuvants depends on the expected time of surgery

** Not recommended

° Lumbar approach with hyperbaric local anaesthetic. With or without high lumbar epidural catheter

Table 5. Outpatient plastic surgery procedures and doses of intrathecal local anesthetics *

Estimated surgery time	Drugs recommended
Up to one hour	Lidocaine + clonidine Lidocaine + fentanyl Articaine + fentanyl Chloroprocaine + fentanyl or clonidine Small doses of PPX + fentanyl or clonidine
One to two hours	PPX + clonidine or fentanyl
Two to four hours	PPX + clonidine or fentanyl PPX + clonidine + fentanyl
More than 4 hours	PPX + clonidine + fentanyl PPX + clonidine + morphine

PPX=Racemic bupivacaine, Levobupivacaine, Ropivacaine, or Mepivacaine

Table 6. Recommended drug combination for spinal anaesthesia according with expected surgery time

7. Adjuvant drugs

Adjuvant drugs for spinal anaesthesia in outpatients and short-stay cases are a usual routine in our daily practice in order to decrease the dose of LAs, facilitate a faster recovery and effective postoperative analgesia. There are numerous receptors which modulate spinal pain response, however, there are only a few drugs for subarachnoid use acting as adjuvants. Adrenaline was the most widely used adjuvant in spinal anaesthesia before the use of neuroaxial opioids. Its use has been questioned because 100-300 μg added to LAs did not prolong spinal anaesthesia, but delays recovery. There are some intrathecal adjuvants that have not been approved to be used in spinal anaesthesia like midazolam, ketamine and neostigmine. They may also improve the quality of block and prolong analgesia. Intrathecal magnesium sulphate mainly potentiates the analgesic action of intrathecal opioids, without significant side effects. A positive impact on spinal analgesia has also been suggested for intrathecal calcium channel blockers, and nonsteroidal anti-inflammatory drugs. Alpha2 agonists and opioids are the most used spinal adjuvants drugs.

Alpha2 agonists. Alpha2 agonists drugs are being increasingly used in critical care and anaesthesia. Beside analgesia and sedation, they also decrease sympathetic tone and attenuate the stress response to anaesthesia and surgery. Historically, adrenaline was the first alpha2 agonist used intrathecally but it is no longer recommended. Clonidine and dexmedetomidine are also members of this group of adjuvant drugs. Their site of action involves specific receptors of the spinal dorsal horn and supraspinaly in the nucleus coereleus in the pons. Spinal injection of clonidine and dexmedetomidine enhance duration and quality of subarachnoid anaesthesia without neurotoxicity. Continuous administration of spinal clonidine in Wistar rats during 14 days failed to demonstrate neurotoxic damage.[88] Erddivanli and coworkers injected male Sprague-Dawley rats [89] with 3 μg and 10 μg of intrathecal dexmedetomidine added to bupivacaine found no apparent pathohistological changes 24 hours after a single injection. In male Kunming mice 1 to 3 μg of dexmedetomidine displayed a robust analgesia via a $\alpha 2$-receptor in a dose dependent manner and no significant pathological impacts on the spinal cord were noticed, with a potential protective effects of lidocaine induced neural cell damage. [90]

Clonidine. Is an alpha2 agonist used in anaesthesia for various purposes. When injected neuroaxialy, it prolongs sensory and motor block, increases sedation and may potentiate hypotension and bradycardia. It has been extensively studied in high (> 150 μg), low (< 150 μg) and small (< 75 μg) doses. Doses of 150, 300 and 450 μg produce dose dependent analgesia, [91] and enhance spinal anaesthesia, with relative hemodynamic stability. Doses of 15 and 30 μg in addition to 11 mg of spinal hyperbaric bupivacaine [92] provide better sensory and motor block compared to bupivacaine alone, but clonidine 30 μg was associated with more incidence and duration of hypotension. Mirivirta et al used 15 μg of clonidine in lateral spinal anesthesia with hyperbaric bupivacaine 5 mg [93] in outpatients undergoing knee arthroscopy reporting intensified spinal lateral anaesthesia without affecting home-readiness. A systematic review [94] including 1,445 patients using a wide variety of spinal clonidine doses as adjuvant to subarachnoid bupivacaine, mepivacaine, prilocaine, or tetracaine found that 15 to 150 μg prolonged in a linear, dose-dependent manner, the time to 2 segment regression (range of means, 14 to 75 minutes) and also delayed the time to regression to L2 (range of means, 11 to 128 minutes). The time to first analgesic request (median 101 minutes, range 35 to 310) and of motor block (median 47 minutes, range 6 to 131) was extended with no relation to dose. There were fewer episodes of intraoperative pain with clonidine (relative risk, 0.24; 95% confidence interval [CI], 0.09-0.64; number needed to treat, 13) but more episodes of arterial hypotension (relative risk, 1.81; 95% CI 1.44-2.28; number needed to harm, 8) without evidence of dose-responsiveness. The risk of bradycardia was unchanged.

The optimal dose of spinal clonidine remains unknown. In our current practice, for short ambulatory procedures we use clonidine 30 to 50 μg added to LA without negative impact on home discharge criteria. For short-stay plastic surgery we use from 75 up to 300 μg of clonidine as adjuvant for any PPX family local anaesthetics.

Dexmedetomidine. Is the newest agent in this group. It was approved by FDA in 1999 for use in humans for analgesia and sedation in the intubated patients at the intensive care settings. It has a α_2/α_1 selectivity ratio which is eight to 10 times higher than that of clonidine. Although it has not been approved for spinal use, there is some research that shows its safety and effectiveness by prolonging time of sensory and motor block of subarachnoid anaesthesia. Kanasi and coworkers [95] compared spinal dexmedetomidine 3 μg versus spinal clonidine 30 μg added to 12 mg subarachnoid bupivacaine versus plain bupivacaine. They found that both alfa2 agonists shorten onset time of motor block and significantly prolonged sensory and motor times. The mean time of sensory regression to the S1 segment was 303 ± 75 minutes in dexmedetomidine patients, 272 ± 38 minutes in those who received clonidine and 190 ± 48 min in control group. The regression of motor block to Bromage 0 was 250 ± 76 minutes in dexmedetomidine group, 216 ± 35 minutes in clonidine cases and 163 ± 47 minutes in control group. The onset and regression times were not significantly different between groups treated with both alfa2 agonists. The mean arterial pressure, heart rate and level of sedation were similar in the three groups intraoperatively and postoperatively. Five μg of dexmedetomidine added to 0.75 isobaric ropivacaine prolonged duration of motor and sensory block, and enhance post operatory analgesia,[96] and significantly prolonged sensory and motor block and reduced demand of rescue analgesics in 24 hours when compared with 25 μg fentanyl and 30 μg clonidine when added to 12.5 mg hyperbaric bupivacaine for spinal anaesthesia.[97] In elderly patients managed with 6 mg 0.5% spinal bupivacaine, the addition of only 3 μg of dexmedetomidine accelerated the blockade onset and prolonged the duration of anaesthesia and postoperative analgesia, although recovery of motor block was affected.[98]

It has been shown that intravenous dexmedetomidine and clonidine significantly prolong bupivacaine spinal anaesthesia, with good sedation effect and hemodynamic stability. In 2003 Rhee et al [99] published the first clinical article with intravenous clonidine to prolong spinal anaesthesia; iv. clonidine 3μg/ kg^{-1} during 10 min immediately after the subarachnoid block or at 50 min after spinal anaesthesia, prolonged significantly duration of motor and sensory block for approximately one hour. In 2007 we found that dexmedetomidine i.v. also improves bupivacaine spinal anaesthesia.[100] In our research we use an i.v. infusion of 1 μg/Kg dexmedetomidine given in 20 min, followed by 0.5 μg/kg/h dexmedetomidine drip until end

http://dx.doi.org/10.5772/58407

of surgery. A comparative group was treated with clonidine 4 μg/kg, given in 20 min i.v. infusion started 20 min after the spinal block, and followed by a 0.9% saline drip until the end of surgery. Sensory block duration was longer in both groups, 208±43.5 and 225±58.8 min respectively, *vs.* placebo group 137±121.9 min (p=0.05). Motor block duration was longer in clonidine than dexmedetomidine (191±49.8 and 172±36.4) *vs.* placebo group (172±36.4) without significative statistical difference. Other authors have confirmed our initial results using i.v. dexmedetomidine doses from 0.25 to 0.5 μg/kg as an initial bolus, followed or not by an infusion of 0.5 μg/kg/h.[101, 102, 103] Two meta-analysis [104,105] showed that i.v. dexmedetomidine prolonged the duration of spinal anaesthesia and improved postoperative analgesia without increasing the incidence of hypotension and adverse events. Transient reversible bradycardia was a mild side effect.

Opioids. Since Yask and Rudy demonstrated that intrathecal opioids produced potent and selective analgesia, neuroaxial opioids are the drugs most used for this purpose. All opioids administered intrathecally will produce some degree of spinally mediated analgesia. The major differences are related to their solubility characteristics and their effect on duration of action, clearance rate, and side effects. Experimental and clinical studies have demonstrated that after their neuroaxial injection, opioid liposolubility is inversely proportional to their spinal selectivity, which is higher for the most water-soluble drugs, morphine and hydromorphone, than for other more lipophilic drugs, such as fentanyl and sufentanyl.[107] Morphine significantly prolongs spinal analgesia and fentanyl and sufentanyl enhance and moderately prolong the sensory block without affecting motor function. Nausea, vomiting, pruritus, and urinary retention are frequent side effects, respiratory depression is seldom observed.

Morphine. Although spinal morphine is the gold standard for opioid neuroaxial post operatory analgesia, it is not the best choice for ambulatory nor short-stay surgery due to a greater incidence of adverse effects that requires cautious patient selection and monitoring. Morphine produces intense analgesia for up to 24-30 hours with doses as low as 100 μg. In our practice we avoid its use in plastic surgery patients.

Fentanyl. Is the most suitable opioid for ambulatory surgery patients. It has the strongest effect at the spinal cord administered spinally or epidurally, producing a short-term analgesia (1-4 hours), which is very helpful in acute postoperative pain. It has been used together with most local anaesthetics in doses from 10 μg up to 25 μg providing selective intra and postoperative analgesia, patient satisfaction, without delaying recovery time.[55,56,60,66,67,107,108,109,110] The most recommended doses are 20 and 25 μg in different outpatient scenarios. Levobupivacaine 3 mg plus 10 μg fentanyl may be used as a suitable alternative to 10 mg lidocaine plus 10 μg fentanyl for subarachnoid anaesthesia of short duration. It achieved a clinically equivalent time for resolution of sensory block, similar intraoperative conditions, and comparable patient satisfaction.[111] The most common side effects are nausea, vomit and itching can be prevented or treated with nalbuphine, droperidol,[112], propofol or ondansetron.

8. Criteria for home discharge

Outpatient plastic surgery patients managed with spinal anaesthesia must meet established home discharge criteria. The goal of these criteria is to discharge patients safely and avoid hospital readmissions due to complications. Pain, nausea, vomiting, and urinary retention are common examples. It is not entirely necessary to fulfill 100% of these home discharge standards, but patients should be warned about the gradual disappearance of spinal anaesthesia side effects, and facilitate easy communication with the surgical unit, the surgeon and anaesthesiologist. These patients require postanaesthetic and appropriate postoperative orders, transportation, and occasional professional company. It is vital that each unit defines its own ambulatory surgery discharge criteria, according to the characteristics and specific needs of their patients.[3,4] Table 7 shows the most common discharge criteria.

Hemodynamic stability	Vital signs return to pre-anaesthetic values is mandatory
Full alertnesss	Patient awake, well oriented. Spinal anaesthesia promotes alertness which facilitates optimal conditions for early home discharge
Permeable digestive tract	Tolerance to solid or liquid intake without nausea or vomiting
Without or mild pain	Controlled postoperative pain (VAS <2/10) with oral analgesics. Spinal anaesthesia with adjuvants provides an extended period of analgesia, it does facilitate early home discharge and reduce analgesics needs.It is desirable to prescribe a combination of opioid and non-opioid analgesics for expected postoperative pain and patient profile.
Spontaneous bladder voiding	This is a controversial requirement. Some centers consider it as mandatory to prevent readmissions for distended bladder. In our practice we do not consider this requirement as essential and the patient knows the remote possibility of urinating difficulties. We avoid the use of intrathecal opioids to reduce this risk.
Ability to walk	Complete regression of motor block is convenient. The patient may try to walk when perianal sensitivity has been recovered, and is able to flex and extend the foot. In some cases it is feasible to discharge without 100% motor recovery.
Headache	While classical PDPH occurs after 2 to 5 days after spinal anaesthesia, there are patients that may develop it in the immediate postoperative period. It is wise to investigate PDPH symptoms with the patient seated or in a standing position.
Others	No surgical bleeding, guaranteed companionship during recovery, transportation and accommodation, do not drive. Keep an established secure communication such as telephone, FAX, e-mail.

Table 7. Home discharge criteria

9. Conclusions

Outpatient and short-stay plastic surgery cases have grown exponentially worldwide. Anaesthesiologists need to provide a safe anaesthesia to these patients who are often subjected

http://dx.doi.org/10.5772/58407

to prolonged surgeries with risks that are higher than expected. Nowadays most cosmetic operations can be done in outpatient and short-stay facilities thanks to advances in anaesthesia. Although most anesthesiologists use general anesthesia for these procedures, regional anesthesia techniques have demonstrated certain advantages such as better pain control, attenuation of the surgical stress response, preserves perioperative immune function, better preservation of oxygenation and lung residual functional capacity, improved visceral vascular flow, less bleeding, early recovery of postoperative ileum, and reduced venous thrombotic disease and pulmonary embolism.

Spinal anaesthesia is a simple technique, with a small volume of drugs producing profound anaesthesia and analgesia, and is devoid of systemic pharmacologic side effects. There are many choices of LAs for outpatient and short-stay spinal anaesthesia; for ultra short procedures the best choice are procaine, articaine or lidocaine. For intermediate duration procedures small doses of intermediate duration LAs, or even lidocaine can be used. For longer procedures bupivacaine, levobupivacaine, and ropivacaine are excellent agents. Addition of adjuvant drugs to LAs enhance subarachnoid anaesthesia with better recovery according with expected surgical time, low incidence of side effects or complications, and longer postoperative analgesia. Clonidine and dexmedetomidine accelerate the onset and prolong the duration of spinal anaesthesia and analgesia.

Severe complications after spinal anesthesia are exceedingly rare; cardiac arrest, meningitis, intracranial subdural hematoma, spinal epidural hematoma, TNS and cauda equina syndrome. Patients should be informed in detail regarding the incidence, severity, and outcome of these complications.

Author details

Víctor M. Whizar-Lugo[1], Juan C. Flores-Carrillo[2], Susana Preciado-Ramírez[3], Jaime Campos-León[4] and Víctor Silva[5]

1 Anesthesiology, Pain Medicine and Critical Care Medicine, Investigador Asociado C, Institutos Nacionales de Salud, Anestesiología y Medicina del Dolor, Centro Médico del Noroeste, Tijuana BC, México

2 Anesthesiology and Critical Care Medicine, Centro Médico del Noroeste, Tijuana BC, México

3 Anesthesiology, Fundación Médica Sur, Ciudad de México, México

4 Campos-León Plastic Surgery Center, Tijuana, México

5 Anesthesiology and Pain Medicine, Hospital Universitario Dr. José Eleuterio González, Monterrey NL, México

References

[1] Shapiro FE. Anesthesia for outpatient cosmetic surgery. Curr Opin Anaesthesiol. 2008;21:704-10.

[2] Hafezi F, Naghibzadeh B, Nouhi AH, Salimi A, Naghibzadeh G, Mousavi SJ. Epidural anesthesia as a thromboembolic prophylaxis modality in plastic surgery. Aesthet Surg J. 2011;31:821-4.

[3] Whizar-Lugo VM, Cisneros-Corral R, Reyes-Aveleyra MA, Campos-León J, Shakhov A. Anestesia subaracnoidea en cirugía plástica ambulatoria. Anest Mex 2008;20:23-33.

[4] Whizar-Lugo V, Cisneros-Corral R, Reyes-Aveleyra MA, Campos-León J. Domínguez J. Anesthesia for plastic surgery procedures in previously morbidly obese patients. Anest Mex 2009;21:186-193.

[5] Dini GM, Ferreira MC, Albuquerque LG, Ferreira LM. How safe is thromboprophylaxis in abdominoplasty? Plast Reconstr Surg. 2012;130:851e-857e.

[6] Neaman KC, Hansen JE.Analysis of complications from abdominoplasty: a review of 206 cases at a university hospital. Ann Plast Surg. 2007;58:292-8.

[7] Pannucci CJ, Bailey SH, Dreszer G, et al. Validation of the Caprini risk assessment model in plastic and reconstructive surgery patients.J Am Coll Surg. 2011;212:105-12.

[8] Rawal N, Holmström B. The combined spinal--epidural technique. Best Pract Res Clin Anaesthesiol. 2003;17:347-64.

[9] Kodeih MG, Al-Alami AA, Atiyeh BS, Kanazi GE. Combined spinal epidural anesthesia in an asthmatic patient undergoing abdominoplasty. Plast Reconstr Surg. 2009;123:118e-120e.

[10] Svetlov VA, Kozlov SP, Vashchinskaia TV, Sarkisova NG. Subarachnoidal anesthesia: the limits of its potentials. Anesteziol Reanimatol. 1999;5:38-44.

[11] Whizar LV, Carrada PS, Cisneros CR, Cortes GC, Solar LC. Migración subaracnoidea del catéter o del anestésico durante anestesia epidural-espinal combinada. Informe de un caso. Rev Mex Anest 1997;20:91-5.

[12] Dean HP. Discussion on the relative value of inhalation and injection methods of inducing anaesthesia. Br Med J 1907;5:869-77.

[13] Lemmon WT. A method for continuous spinal anesthesia: A preliminary report. Ann Surg. 1940;111:141-4.

[14] Hurley RJ, Lambert DH. Continuous spinal anesthesia with a microcatheter technique: preliminary experience. Anesth Analg. 1990;70:97-102.

[15] Lux EA. Continuous spinal anesthesia for lower limb surgery: a retrospective analysis of 1212 cases. Local Reg Anesth. 2012;5:63-7.

[16] Dhami LD. Liposuction. Indian J Plast Surg. 2008;41(Suppl):S27-40.

[17] Whizar LV, Cisneros CR, Reyes AMA, Ontiveros MP. Combined lumbar spinal-epidural anaesthesia (CLSEA) with hyperbaric 0.75% ropivacaine plus clonidine for breast and abdominal-pelvic plastic surgery. An open trial. WCA Paris, France. 2004;CD231.

[18] Di Cianni S, Rossi M, Casati A, Cocco C, Fanelli G. Spinal anesthesia: an evergreen technique. Acta Biomed. 2008;79:9-17.

[19] Liu SS.Optimizing spinal anesthesia for ambulatory surgery. Reg Anesth. 1997;22:500-10.

[20] Casati A, Vinciguerra F. Intrathecal anesthesia. Curr Opin Anaesthesiol. 2002;15:543-51.

[21] Urmey WF. Spinal anaesthesia for outpatient surgery. Best Pract Res Clin Anaesthesiol. 2003;17:335-46.

[22] Pitkänen MT, Aromaa U, Cozanitis DA, Förster JG. Serious complications associated with spinal anaesthesia in Finlad from 2000 to 2009. Acta Anaesthesiol Scand. 2013;57:553-64.

[23] Pollard JB.Cardiac arrest during spinal anesthesia: common mechanisms and strategies for prevention. Anesth Analg. 2001;92:252-6.

[24] Limongi JA, Lins RS.Cardiopulmonary arrest in spinal anesthesia. Rev Bras Anestesiol. 2011;61:110-20.

[25] Auroy Y, Narchi P, Messiah A, Litt L, Rouvier B, Samii K. Serious complications related to regional anesthesia: results of a prospective survey in France. Anesthesiology. 1997;87:479-86.

[26] Takenami T, Yagishita S, Asato F, Arai M, Hoka S. Intrathecal lidocaine causes posterior root axonal degeneration near entry into the spinal cord in rats. Reg Anesth Pain Med. 2002;27:58-67.

[27] Schneider M, Ettllin T, Kaufmann M. et al. Transient neurologic toxicity after hyperbaric subarachnoid anesthesia with 5% lidocaine. Anest Analg 1993:76;1154-57.

[28] Takenami T, Yagishita S, Nara Y, et al. Spinal procaine is less neurotoxic than mepivacaine, prilocaine and bupivacaine in rats. Reg Anesth Pain Med. 2009;34:189-95.

[29] Takenami T, Yagishita S, Murase S, et al. Neurotoxicity of intrathecally administered bupivacaine involves the posterior roots/posterior white matter and is milder than lidocaine in rats. Reg Anesth Pain Med. 2005;30:464-72.

[30] Takenami T, Wang G, Nara Y, et al. Intrathecally administered ropivacaine is less neurotoxic than procaine, bupivacaine, and levobupivacaine in a rat spinal model. Can J Anaesth. 2012;59:456-65.

[31] Zhong Z, Qulian G, Yuan Z, Wangyuan Z, Zhihua S. Repeated intrathecal administration of ropivacaine causes neurotoxicity in rats. Anaesth Intensive Care. 2009;37:929-36.

[32] Rätsch G, Niebergall H, Hauenstein L, et al. Spinal anaesthesia in day-case surgery. Optimisation of procedures. Anaesthesist 2007;56:322-27.

[33] Carrada PS, Whizar LV, Pérez OA, Cabrera MN. Incidencia de cefalea postraquia en pacientes jóvenes. Estudio doble ciego, comparativo con Atraucan 26, Quincke 26 y Whitacre 27. Rev Mex Anest 1997;20:3-10.

[34] Reina MA, De Leon O, Lopez A, De Andres J, Martin S, Mora M. An in vitro study of dural lesions produced by 25-gauge Quincke and Whitacre needles evaluated by scanning electron microscopy. Reg Anesth Pain Med 2000;25:393-402.

[35] Fettes PDW, Jansson JR, Wildsmith JAW. Failed spinal anaesthesia: mechanisms, management, and prevention. Brit J Anaesth 2009;102:739-48.

[36] Abouleish E. How to proceed following a °failed spinal°. Anesthesiology 1992;76:476-7.

[37] Drasner K, Rigler ML. Repeat injection after a failed spinal: At times, a potentially unsafe practice. Anesthesiology 1991;75:713-4.

[38] Aldrete A. Neurologic deficits and arachnoiditis following neuroaxial anesthesia. Acta Anaesthesiol Scand 2003;47:3-12.

[39] Castillo J, Santiveri X, Escolano F, et al. Incidencia de hematomas espinales con compresión medular relacionados con anestesias neuroaxiales en Cataluña. Rev Esp Anestesiol Reanim. 2007;54:591-5.

[40] Horlocker TT, Wedel DJ, Rowlingson JC, et al. Regional anesthesia in the patient receiving antithrombotic or thrombolytic therapy: American Society of Regional Anesthesia and Pain Medicine Evidence-Based Guidelines (Third Edition). Reg Anesth Pain Med. 2010;35:64-101.

[41] Förster JG, Rosenberg PH. Revival of old local anesthetics for spinal anesthesia in ambulatory surgery. Curr Opin Anaesthesiol. 2011;24:633-7.

[42] Hendriks MP, de Weert CJ, Snoeck MM, Hu HP, Pluim MA, Gielen MJ. Plain articaine or prilocaine for spinal anaesthesia in day-case knee arthroscopy: a double-blind randomized trial. Br J Anaesth. 2009;102:259-63.

[43] Whizar LV, Carrada PS. Ropivacaína: una novedosa alternativa en anestesia regional. Rev Mex Anest 1999;22:122-152.

[44] Wille M. Intrathecal use of ropivacaine: a review. Acta Anaesthesiol Belg 2004;55:251-9.

[45] Sanansilp V, Trivate T, Chompubai P, et al. Clinical characteristics of spinal levobupivacaine: hyperbaric compared with isobaric solution. ScientificWorld Journal. 2012;2012:169076.

[46] Zaric D, Pace NL. Transient neurologic symptoms (TNS) following spinal anaesthesia with lidocaine versus other local anaesthetics. Cochrane Database Syst Rev. 2009 Apr 15;[2]:CD003006.

[47] Waxler B, Mondragon SA, Patel SN, Nedumgottil K. Intrathecal lidocaine and sufentanil shorten postoperative recovery after outpatient rectal surgery. Can J Anaesth 2004;51:680-4.

[48] Frey K, Holman S, Mikat-Stevens M et al. The recovery profile of hyperbaric spinal anesthesia with lidocaine, tetracaine, and bupivacaine. Reg Anesth Pain Med 1998;23:159-163.

[49] Pawlowski J, Orr K, Kim KM, Pappas AL, Sukhani R, Jellish WS. Anesthetic and recovery profiles of lidocaine versus mepivacaine for spinal anesthesia in patients undergoing outpatient orthopedic arthroscopic procedures. J Clin Anesth. 2012;24:109-15.

[50] Kallio H, Snall EV, Luode T, Rosenberg PH. Hyperbaric articaine for day-case spinal anaesthesia. Br J Anaesth. 2006;97:704-9.

[51] Timmerman L, van Dongen EP, Tromp E, Andriessen EJ, Kerkvliet CT, Knibbe CA. Articaine and lidocaine for spinal anaesthesia in day case surgery. Reg Anesth Pain Med. 2007;32 Suppl 1:9.

[52] Snoeck M. Articaine: a review of its use for local and regional anesthesia. Local Reg Anesth 2012;5:23-33.

[53] Malinovsky JM. Is 4% Articaine suitable for spinal anesthesia. Eur J Anesthesiol. 2012;29:5-6.

[54] Hendriks MP, de Weert CJ, Snoeck MM, Hu HP, Pluim MA, Gielen MJ. Plain articaine or prilocaine for spinal anaesthesia in day-case knee arthroscopy: a double-blind randomized trial. Br J Anaesth. 2009;102:259-63.

[55] Kairaluoma P, Bachmann M, Kallio H, Rosenberg P, Pere P. Hyperbaric articaine with or without fentanyl in spinal anaesthesia: patient and observer blinded comparison. Acta Anaesthesiol Scand. 2013;57:118-25.

[56] Bachmann M, Pere P, Kairaluoma P, Rosenberg PH, Kallio H. Randomised comparison of hyperbaric articaine and hyperbaric low-dose bupivacaine along with fentanyl inspinal anaesthesia for day-case inguinal herniorrhaphy. Eur J Anaesthesiol. 2012;29:22-7.

[57] Lee YY, Ngan Kee WD, Fong SY, Liu JT, Gin T. The median effective dose of bupivacaine, levobupivacaine, and ropivacaine after intrathecal injection in lower limb surgery. Anesth Analg. 2009;109:1331-4.

[58] Nair GS, Abrishami A, Lermitte J, Chung F. Systematic review of spinal anaesthesia using bupivacaine for ambulatory knee arthroscopy. Br J Anaesth. 2009;102:307-15.

[59] Casati A, Cappelleri G, Fanelli G, et al. Regional anaesthesia for outpatient knee arthroscopy: a randomized clinical comparison of two different anaesthetic techniques. Acta Anaesthesiol Scand 2000;44:543-7.

[60] Unal D, Ozdogan L, Ornek HD, et al. Selective spinal anaesthesia with low-dose bupivacaine and bupivacaine+fentanyl in ambulatory arthroscopic knee surgery. J Pak Med Assoc. 2012;62:313-8.

[61] Marin R, Frigon CH, Chrétien A, Tétraul JP. Onset of spinal block is more rapid with isobaric than hyperbaric bupivacaine. Can J Anesth 2000;47:43-6.

[62] Vasconcelos Filho Pde O, Posso Ide P, Capelozzi M, Capelozzi VL. Comparison of histologic spinal cord and neurologic changes in guinea pigs after subarachnoid block with large volumes of racemic bupivacaine, 50% enantiomeric excess bupivacaine (S75-R25], and levobupivacaine. Rev Bras Anestesiol. 2008;58:234-45.

[63] Hamurtekin E, Fitzsimmons BL, Shubayev VI, et al. Evaluation of spinal toxicity and long-term spinal reflex function after intrathecal levobupivaciane in the neonatal rat. Anesthesiology. 2013;119:142-55.

[64] Burke D, Kennedy S, Bannister J. Spinal anesthesia with 0.5% S(-)-bupivacaine for elective lower limb surgery. Reg Anesth Pain Med 1999;24:519-523.

[65] Onur O, Sibel AM, Mustafa A, Mehmet Y.Comparison of the effects of intrathecal different dosage of levobupivacaine in elective day-case arthroscopy of the knee. Middle East J Anesthesiol. 2010;20:703-8.

[66] de Santiago J, Santos-Yglesias J, Giron J, Montes de Oca F, Jimenez A, Diaz P. Low-dose 3 mg levobupivacaine plus 10 microg fentanyl selective spinal anesthesia for gynecological outpatient laparoscopy. Anesth Analg. 2009;109:1456-61.

[67] Girgin NK, Gurbet A, Turker G, et al. The combination of low-dose levobupivacaine and fentanyl for spinal anaesthesia in ambulatory inguinal herniorrhaphy. J Int Med Res. 2008;36:1287-92.

[68] Sanansilp V, Trivate T, Chompubai P, et al. Clinical characteristics of spinal levobupivacaine: hyperbaric compared with isobaric solution. ScientificWorldJournal. 2012;2012:169076.

[69] Erdil F, Bulut S, Demirbilek S, Gedik E, Gulhas N, Ersoy MO. The effects of intrathecal levobupivacaine and bupivacaine in the elderly. Anaesthesia. 2009;64:942-6.

[70] Gozdemir M, Muslu B, Sert H, et al. Transient neurological symptoms after spinal anaesthesia with levobupivacaine 5 mg/ml or lidocaine 20 mg/ml. Acta Anaesthesiol Scand. 2010;54:59-64.

[71] Martínez-Gallegos N, Reyes-Aveleyra MA, Whizar-Lugo VM. Síndrome de irritación transitoria secundario a levobupivacaína 0.65% subaracnoidea. Informe de un caso. Anest Mex 2006;18:96-100.

[72] López-Soriano F, Lajarín B, Rivas F, Verdú JM, López-Robles J. Ropivacaína hiperbárica subaracnoidea en cirugía ambulatoria: estudio comparativo con bupivacaína hiperbárica. Rev Esp Anestesiol Reanim 2002;49:71-5.

[73] Buckenmaier CC 3rd, Nielsen KC, Pietrobon R, et al. Small-dose intrathecal lidocaine versus ropivacaine for anorectal surgery in an ambulatory setting. Anesth Analg. 2002;95:1253-7.

[74] Fanelli G, Danelli G, Zasa M, Baciarello M, Di Cianni S, Leone S. Intrathecal ropivacaine 5 mg/ml for outpatient knee arthroscopy: a comparison with lidocaine 10 mg/ml. Acta Anaesthesiol Scand. 2009;53:109-15.

[75] Taspinar V, Sahin A, Donmez NF, et al. Low-dose ropivacaine or levobupivacaine walking spinal anesthesia in ambulatory inguinal herniorrhaphy. J Anesth. 2011;25:219-24.

[76] Gautier PE, DeKock M, Van Steenberge A. Intrathecal ropivacaine for ambulatory surgery: A comparison between intrathecal bupivacaine and intrathecal ropivacaine for knee arthroscopy. Anesthesiology 1999;91:1239-1245.

[77] Whizar-Lugo VM, Martínez Gallegos N, Domínguez J. Sobredosis intratecal accidental de 30mg de ropivacaína al 1%. Informe de un paciente. Anest Mex 2007;19:41-6.

[78] YaDeau JT, Liguori GA, Zayas VM. The incidence of transient neurologic symptoms after spinal anesthesia with mepivacaine. Anesth Analg. 2005;101:661-5.

[79] Pawlowski J, Sukhani R, Pappas AL et al. The anesthetic and recovery profile of two doses [60 and 80 mg) of plain mepivacaine for ambulatory spinal anesthesia. Anesth Analg. 2000;91:580-4.

[80] Pawlowski J, Orr K, Kim KM, Pappas AL, Sukhani R, Jellish WS. Anesthetic and recovery profiles of lidocaine versus mepivacaine for spinal anesthesia in patients undergoing outpatient orthopedic arthroscopic procedures. J Clin Anesth. 2012;24:109-15.

[81] O'Donnell D, Manickam B, Perlas A, et al. Spinal mepivacaine with fentanyl for outpatient knee arthroscopy surgery: a randomized controlled trial. Can J Anaesth. 2010;57:32-8.

[82] Kopacz DJ. Spinal 2-chloroprocaine: minimum effective dose. Reg Anesth Pain Med. 2005;30:36-42.

[83] Hejtmanek MR, Pollock JE. Chloroprocaine for spinal anesthesia: a retrospective analysis. Acta Anaesthesiol Scand. 2011;55:267-72.

[84] Förster JG, Rosenberg PH, Harilainen A, Sandelin J, Pitkänen MT. Chloroprocaine 40 mg produces shorter spinal block than articaine 40 mg in day-case knee arthroscopy patients. Acta Anaesthesiol Scand. 2013;57:911-9.

[85] Goldblum E, Atchabahian A.The use of 2-chloroprocaine for spinal anaesthesia. Acta Anaesthesiol Scand. 2013;57:545-52.

[86] Johnson ME, Swanson JW. Procaine spinal neurotoxicity. Anesthesiology. 2008;109:349-51.

[87] Hodgson PS, Liu SS, Batra MS, Gras TW, Pollock JE, Neal JM. Procaine compared to lidocaine for incidence of transient neurologic symptoms. Reg Anesth Pain Med 2000;25:218-22.

[88] Guevara-López U, Aldrete JA, Covarrubias-Gómez A, Hernández-Pando RE, López-Muñoz FJ. Absence of histological changes after the administration of a continuous intrathecal clonidine in Wistar rats. Pain Pract. 2009;9:122-9.

[89] Erdivanli B, Altun M, Sezen OK, Colakoğlu SA. Anti-nociceptive, analgesic and pathohistological effects of intrathecal dexmedetomidine and bupivacaine in rats. Rev Bras Anestesiol. 2013;63:183-7.

[90] Zhang H, Zhou F, Li C, et al. Molecular mechanisms underlying the analgesic property of intrathecal dexmedetomidine and its neurotoxicity evaluation: an in vivo and in vitro experimental study. PLoS One. 2013;8:e55556.

[91] Filos KS, Goudas LC, Patroni O, Polyzou V. Hemodynamic and analgesic profile after intrathecal clonidine in humans. A dose-response study. Anesthesiology 1994;81:591-601.

[92] Thakur A, Bhardwaj M, Kaur K, Dureja J, Hooda S, Taxak S. Intrathecal clonidine as an adjuvant to hyperbaric bupivacaine in patients undergoing inguinal herniorrhaphy: A randomized double-blinded study. J Anaesthesiol Clin Pharmacol. 2013;29:66-70.

[93] Merivirta R, Kuusniemi K, Jaakkola P, Pihlajamäki K, Pitkänen M.Unilateral spinal anaesthesia for outpatient surgery: a comparison between hyperbaric bupivacaine and bupivacaine-clonidine combination. Acta Anaesthesiol Scand. 2009;53:788-93.

[94] Elia N, Culebras X, Mazza C, Schiffer E, Tramèr MR. Clonidine as an adjuvant to intrathecal local anesthetics for surgery: systematic review of randomized trials. Reg Anesth Pain Med. 2008;33:159-67.

[95] Kanazi GE, Aouad MT, Jabbour-Khoury SI, et al. Effect of low-dose dexmedetomidine or clonidine on the characteristics of bupivacaine spinal block. Acta Anaesthesiol Scand. 2006;50:222-7.

[96] Gupta R, Bogra J, Verma R, Kohli M, Kushwaha JK, Kumar S. Dexmedetomidine as an intrathecal adjuvant for postoperative analgesia. Indian J Anaesth. 2011;55:347-51.

[97] Mahendru V, Tewari A, Katyal S, Grewal A, Singh MR, Katyal R. A comparison of intrathecal dexmedetomidine, clonidine, and fentanyl as adjuvants of hyperbaric bupivacaine for lower limb surgery: A double blind controlled study. J Anaesthesiol Clin Pharmacol 2013;29:496-502.

[98] Kim JE, Kim NY, Lee HS, Kil HK. Effects of intrathecal dexmedetomidine on low-dose bupivacaine spinal anesthesia in elderly patients undergoing transurethral prostatectomy. Biol Pharm Bull. 2013;36:959-65.

[99] Rhee K, Kang K, Kim J, Jeon Y. Intravenous clonidine prolongs bupivacaine spinal anesthesia. Acta Anaesthesiol Scand. 2003;47:1001-1005.

[100] Whizar-Lugo V, Gómez-Ramírez IA, Cisneros-Corral R, Martínez-Gallegos N. Intravenous dexmedetomidine vs. intravenous clonidine to prolong bupivacaine spinal anesthesia. A double blind study. Anest Mex 2007;19:143-146.

[101] Harsoor S, Rani DD, Yalamuru B, Sudheesh K, Nethra S. Effect of supplementation of low dose intravenous dexmedetomidine on characteristics of spinal anaesthesia with hyperbaric bupivacaine. Indian J Anaesth. 2013;57:265-9.

[102] Jung SH, Lee SK, Lim KJ, et al. The effects of single-dose intravenous dexmedetomidine on hyperbaric bupivacaine spinal anesthesia. J Anesth. 2013;27:380-4.

[103] Al-Mustafa MM, Badran IZ, Abu-Ali HM, Al-Barazangi BA, Massad IM, Al-Ghanem SM. Intravenous dexmedetomidine prolongs bupivacaine spinal analgesia. Middle East J Anesthesiol. 2009;20:225-31.

[104] Abdallah FW, Abrishami A, Brull R. The facilitatory effects of intravenous dexmedetomidine on the duration of spinal anesthesia: a systematic review and meta-analysis. Anesth Analg. 2013;117:271-8.

[105] Niu XY, Ding XB, Guo T, Chen MH, Fu SK, Li Q. Effects of intravenous and intrathecal dexmedetomidine in spinal anesthesia: a meta-analysis. CNS Neurosci Ther. 2013;19:897-904.

[106] Bujedo BM, Santos SG, Azpiazu AU.A review of epidural and intrathecal opioids used in the management of postoperative pain. J Opioid Manag. 2012;8:177-92.

[107] de Santiago J, Santos-Yglesias J, Girón J, Jiménez A, Errando CL. Anestesia subaracnoidea hipobárica a dosis bajas para cirugía anorrectal en posición de navaja: comparación entre levobupivacaína-fentanilo y licocaína-fentanilo. Rev Esp Anestesiol Reanim. 2010;57:565-70.

[108] Chilvers CR, Vaghadia H, Mitchell GW, Merrick PM. Small-dose hypobaric lidocaine-fentanyl spinal anesthesia for short duration outpatient laparoscopy. II. Optimal fentanyl dose. Anesth Analg. 1997;84:65-70.

[109] Kallio H, Snäll EV, Suvanto SJ, et al. Spinal hyperbaric ropivacaine-fentanyl for day-surgery. Reg Anesth Pain Med. 2005;30:48-54.

[110] Girgin NK, Gurbet A, Turker G, et al. The combination of low-dose levobupivacaine and fentanyl for spinal anaesthesia in ambulatory inguinal herniorrhaphy. J Int Med Res. 2008;36:1287-92.

[111] de Santiago J, Santos-Yglesias J, Giron J, Montes de Oca F, Jimenez A, Diaz P. Low-dose 3 mg levobupivacaine plus 10 μg fentanyl selective spinal anesthesia for gynecological outpatient laparoscopy. Anesth Analg. 2009;109:1456-61.

[112] Ben-David B, DeMeo PJ, Lucyk C, Solosko D. Minidose lidocaine-fentanyl spinal anesthesia in ambulatory surgery: prophylactic nalbuphine versus nalbuphine plus droperidol. Anesth Analg. 2002;95:1596-600.

Chapter 4

Spinal Additives in Subarachnoid Anaesthesia for Cesarean Section

Hala M. Goma, Juan C. Flores-Carrillo and
Víctor Whizar-Lugo

Additional information is available at the end of the chapter

http://dx.doi.org/10.5772/58851

1. Introduction

Cesarean section is among the most commonly performed surgeries in women and neuroaxial anaesthesia is the technique of choice for this procedure. Although numerous side effects related to obstetric anaesthesia had been described, [1, 2, 3, 4] subarachnoid anaesthesia has a clear tendency to be used more often than epidural and combined spinal-epidural technique. It is safe, easy to perform, effective, low failure rate, no systemic local anaesthetic toxicity, inexpensive, prevents aspiration pneumonia, and has a high rate of maternal satisfaction. [5, 6, 7] Produces a deep anaesthesia, inhibits the stress response to surgery, blunts the autonomic and somatic responses to pain, and facilitate breathing, coughing, sighing and early ambulation [8, 9] Finally, efferent sympathetic blockade results in increased blood flow to the blocked area resulting in better wound healing. It also reduces the risk of deep vein thrombosis and thromboembolism.

The main limitations of spinal anaesthesia are its short duration of action and do not provide prolonged postoperative analgesia when it is performed only with local anaesthetics. Adding adjuvants drugs to intrathecal local anaesthetics improves quality and duration of spinal blockade, and prolongs postoperative analgesia. It is also possible to reduce dose of local anaesthetics, as well as total amount of systemic postoperative analgesics. Several spinal adjuvants have been used to improve spinal anaesthesia quality and to prolong postsurgical analgesia. Intrathecal opioids are the most commonly utilized; fentanyl and sufentanil improve neuroaxial anaesthesia, decrease trans operative pain and moderately prolong sensory block, while morphine prolongs postoperative analgesia. Alpha2 adrenergic agonists clonidine and dexmedetomidine shorten onset of action, and prolong duration of spinal anaesthesia.

Ketamine, midazolam, neostigmine, magnesium sulphate and others spinal drugs are still under investigation.

This chapter is an up to date of spinal additives currently used to enhance subarachnoid anaesthesia for cesarean section and to produce subarachnoid postcesarean analgesia.

2. Spinal additives drugs for cesarean delivery

The use of subarachnoid additives in spinal anaesthesia for cesarean section has two main objectives: to enhance spinal block and to produce effective and prolonged postoperative analgesia. Reducing the dose of local anaesthetics used in spinal anaesthesia can decrease some of the side effects such as maternal hypotension, high spinal block, and prolonged motor block. By inducing better analgesia after cesarean section with intrathecal additives, the recently given birth mother is better able to take care of her newborn, which immediately improves mother-baby relationship, decreases prelacteal feeds (feeding any other substance before first breastfeeding), which is closely related to urban residency, first-time motherhood, and cesarean delivery. Prelacteal feed has been reported as high as 26.5%. It has several harmful effects on the mother-newborn binomia. [10, 11] Immediate proper breast feeding even favor neonatal analgesia for minimum invasive procedures like heel prick. [12]

Postoperative pain after cesarean section is common and more intense compared to postvaginal delivery pain. [13] When this kind of pain is not prevented nor treated properly, it can evolve to chronic pain which means a serious health problem. [14] Therefore, intrathecal adjuvants play an important role not only in maternal analgesia, but in the future of the newborn.

There are several adjuvant drugs used to enhance spinal anaesthesia; morphine is the most frequently used and also many other opioid agonists such fentanyl, sufentanyl, hydromorphone, diamorphine, and meperidine have been well studied and are part of our daily armamentarium in this clinical scenario, as are some non-opioid drugs such clonidine. There is a heterogeneous group including midazolam, neostigmine, magnesium, that needs more research before they can be part of daily use as intrathecal adjuvants for C-section anaesthesia.

Table 1 summarizes the most commonly used spinal additives and some drugs under clinical research in parturients undergoing cesarean delivery with spinal anaesthesia.

3. Spinal opioids

Opioids are the most commonly used analgesics to treat perioperative pain. Since the isolation of morphine in 1804 by Friedrich Sertürner, a pharmacist´s apprentice in Germany, morphine became widely used after 1815. Since then, a large number of opioids have been developed modifying the 4, 5-epoxymorphinan ring structure. Opioids have a narrow therapeutic index with a large inter patient analgesic response variability; from poor analgesia to dangerous side effects.

Morphine was the first spinal drug used to relieve pain, [15] Pert and Snyder [16] discovered the opioid receptors in 1973, and three years after Yaskh and Rudy working at Yale published their famous article entitled *Analgesia mediated by a direct spinal action of narcotics*, [17] which encouraged animal and clinical research for the use of opioids and other neuroaxial additives.

Intrathecal opioids bind to opioid receptors localized in laminae I and II at the spinal dorsal horn reducing nociceptive transmission. Opioids with high lipid solubility and low pKa results in a extremely potent analgesic effect, rapid onset and short duration of action, conversely opioids with diminished lipophilicity such is morphine, have a slow onset and prolonged analgesia. Pharmacokinetically, subarachnoid injection of opioids follows a complex multi compartmental model influenced by opioid properties and cerebro spinal fluid (CSF) dynamics. From the lumbar CSF they move inside the spinal cord binding dorsal horn opiate receptors and also enter the bloodstream through the posterior radicular artery. Spinal opioids also penetrate the dura mater into the epidural cavity and hence can reach the venous plexus of Baston and reach the systemic circulation. They can also move in a cephalad-caudal direction as a drug bulk flow. [18] This rostral migration is probably the most important factor to explain the side effects of opioids, especially deleterious properties of morphine. There are other possible sites where spinal opioids act to produce local anaesthetic effects blocking nerve conduction, [19] or by reducing the release of GABA and glycine by a calcium independent process from dorsal horn neurons. [20]

After local anaesthetics, opioids are the most commonly used drugs by this route providing segmental analgesia. Clinicians have used them for more than 30 years in anaesthesia, for acute pain, postoperative analgesia, and to treat cancer pain. [21, 22] Although spinal opioids are used frequently, there are many unresolved disputes on the neurotoxicity of opioids injected into the subarachnoid space. [23, 24, 25, 26]

In obstetrics patients, neuroaxial opioids use is a significant therapy for labour pain, in cesarean section anaesthesia, and for postoperative pain. A very small dose of almost any opioid delivered into the lumbar spinal space provides significant pain relief with virtually no risk to mother or the fetus-neonate.

Morphine. It is the basic reference opioid to which all analgesics of its kind are compared. It is a phenanthrene derivative, the prototypical agonist opiate at mu and kappa opioid receptors. Has a benzene ring with a phenolic hydroxyl group at position 3 and an alcohol hydroxyl group at position 6 and at the nitrogen atom. Its chemical formula is $C_{17}H_{19}NO_3$. This opioid can be administered by mouth, intravenously, intramuscular, subcutaneously, rectally, intranasal, and through the neuraxial route. Has a significant amount first-pass liver metabolism and about 40 to 50% of the absorbed morphine reach the central nervous system. Most morphine is eliminated by the kidneys. Its poor lipid solubility-a physical characteristic that favors its behavior when injected into the intrathecal space-producing slow analgesic onset with long duration and rostral migration that facilitates some of its side effects such as pruritus, emesis, hypothermia, and respiratory depression. [27, 28]

Although there are places where spinal opioids in obstetrics are not routinely used, [29] at present time, neuraxial morphine is considered as the gold standard to treat pain after C-section and has become a conventional practice in many countries. It is mentioned in textbooks on obstetric and neuroaxial anesthesia [30, 31, 32] as a conventional method. Most authors have reported that 100 to 200 μg of spinal morphine plus regular or low doses of a PPX local anaesthetic or lidocaine are enough to provide an excellent block, high quality postcesarean analgesia, decreased needs of rescue postoperative analgesics, with few side effects. [33-37]

Weigl and coworkers [38] compared intrathecal morphine 100 μg versus spinal fentanyl 25 μg added to 0.5% hyperbaric bupivacaine 7.5 to 15 mg in 60 parturients. Intrathecal morphine drastically prolonged the time for first rescue analgesic, and also reduce postoperative meperidine [47 mg versus 130 mg) when compared to fentanyl. Itch was more often observed in patients treated whit morphine. There was no significant difference in the incidence of postoperative nausea and vomiting between both groups. There were few patients in the morphine group who required additional intravenous opioids during surgery. Bejar et al from Argentina [39] demonstrated that intrathecal morphine 100 μg were better than systemic morphine, although the former had more incidence of itching. In a Brazilian study [40] the authors found that 50 μg of intrathecal morphine produced equal analgesia after cesarean section as 100 μg, but with less incidence of pruritus. Cortes-Blanco et al from México [36], compared morphine 100 μg versus 200 μg added to intrathecal ropivacaine 15 mg in 80 women undergoing cesarean delivery. The analgesic effect lasted 24 to 30 hours, with a low need of postoperative rescue analgesic; ketorolac was used in equal dose in both groups ($p>0.05$]. However side effects were more frequent in those women receiving morphine 200 μg: pruritus 30% versus 55%, nausea 10% versus 30%, and vomiting 5% versus 12.5%. The authors recommended 100 μg as the ideal dose in Mexican parturients undergoing C-section.

Morphine can be coadministered with sufentanil. Draisci et al [41] compared spinal administration of morphine 150 μg plus sufentanil 5 μg versus spinal sufentanil 5 μg plus a single subcutaneous morphine 10 mg in 64 pregnant women undergoing elective cesarean under spinal anaesthesia with hyperbaric bupivacaine 10 mg. Both groups received 1 g acetaminophen every 6 hours and intravenous tramadol was used if VAS was superior to 4. Coadministration of two opioids resulted in prolonged analgesia, less need of tramadol, and less incidence of nausea and no difference in pruritus incidence. Using a combination of spinal morphine 100 μg plus sufentanil 2.5 μg, Bouvet et al [42] determined that the ED_{50} and ED_{95} of intrathecal levobupivacaine is 12.9 mg. For less levobupivacaine dose, the authors recommended to use spinal-epidural combined technique for C-section anaesthesia.

Notwithstanding the multiple investigations to determine the ideal dose, a recent study questioned the best dose of intrathecal morphine for postcesarean analgesia. Wong and coworkers [43] compared the most used doses; 100 versus 200 μg and concluded that the higher dose produce better analgesia but with more nausea, so morphine dosing has to be based on patient preference for analgesia versus emesis.

Recently, in order to avoid spinal morphine side effects, some authors compared ultrasound guided tranversus abdominis plane block versus intrathecal morphine; although ultrasound-guided transversus abdominis plane block is an effective method to supply pain relief after cesarean delivery, 100 μg and 200 μg subarachnoid morphine provided superior analgesia, but emesis and itching were more frequent. This block could be a reasonable alternative when morphine cannot be used. [44, 45]

Hydromorphone. Also known as dihydromorphinone, is a semi-synthetic opioid widely used to treat pain. It is 5 to 11.1 times more potent than morphine, highly soluble in water, with intermediate lipid solubility. The chemical name is 4, 5α-epoxy-3-hydroxy-17-methylmorphinan-6-one hydrochloride, with a molecular formula $C_{17}H_{19}NO_3$ and molecular weight 285.33766. Has a similar pharmacokinetics and duration of action than morphine, is extensively metabolized by the liver to hydromorphone-3-glucoronide with no analgesic effects, 62% of the oral dose is eliminated by this gland on the first pass. Hydromorphone cross the blood brain barrier and reach concentrations in the CNS faster than morphine. Is better tolerated in patients with kidney failure due to a lack of an active metabolite, but its half life can increase to as much as 40 hours. [28, 46]

In a retrospective research, Rauch [47] found that 100 μg of spinal hydromorphone produced a comparable onset of pain relief to 25 μg of subarachnoid fentanyl, with a prolonged analgesia (p<.001] and proposed this opioid as a substitute of intrathecal morphine. Beatty et al [48] compared intrathecal hydromorphone 40 μg versus intrathecal morphine 100 μg in 114 parturients undergoing cesarean section. They found no statistical differences regarding opioid related side effects, rescue analgesics needs or postoperative pain intensity during the first 24 hours. In non obstetric patients [49] nausea is related significantly in a dose-dependent manner. In patients with known allergy to intrathecal morphine, hydromorphone can be used spinally with better analgesic results. [50]

Diamorphine. Also known as heroin, is an pure agonist opioid analgesic 1.5 to 2 times more potent than morphine. In 1874 Charles Write boiled morphine and created heroin. Its chemical name is 4, 5-Epoxy-17-methylmorphinan-3, 6-diyldiacetate hydrochloride monohydrate or [5α, 6α)-7, 8-Didehydro-4, 5-epoxy-17-methylmorphinan-3, 6-diol diacetate (ester), with a molecular formula $C_{21}H_{23}NO_5$. After oral ingest, diamorphine undergoes extensive liver first pass metabolism via deacetylation, transforming into a 6-monoacetylmorphine and morphine. Injected diamorphine, promptly cross the blood-brain barrier and is transformed into morphine by deacetylation, acting over the μ opioid receptors. This opioid can be given by the same routes as morphine in approximately half dose. Its high liposolubility [200 times more liposoluble than morphine) is against rostral migration, consequently reduces the possibility of side effects due to its action on the CNS, especially late respiratory depression. Diamorphine is associated with more euphoria than morphine. [51, 52] This opioid is used for the treatment of pain; severe physical trauma, myocardial infarction, post-surgical pain, and chronic pain, including end-stage cancer and other painful terminal illnesses. Although diamorphine is used for the cure of pain, it is also used illegally by addicts. [51]

Diamorphine had been used neuroaxialy for intraoperative and postcesarean analgesia. Epidural 5 mg produces similar analgesia to 250 μg injected into the subarachnoid space, but with less emesis. [52] Equal doses of diamorphine and intrathecal morphine produce similar postcesarean analgesia but the former has lower frequency and intensity of emesis and pruritus, which is attributed to its greater lipophilicity. [53] Most studies have compared intrathecal doses from 125 up to 375 μg, with similar analgesic results, but a wide outcome regarding incidence of pruritus, nausea and vomit. [54] In a double blind randomized controlled investigation Wrench and coworkers [55] compared spinal diamorphine 0, 100, 200, and 300 μg added to spinal block and systemic diclofenac-paracetamol plus subcutaneous diamorphine for breakthrough pain. They found that 300 μg resulted in better analgesia, but a dose related increase in the incidence of pruritus. In this study, nausea and vomit did not have a dose dependent effect. Spinal diamorphine 300 μg was comparable to intrathecal fentanyl 20 μg regarding needs of intraoperative analgesics supplementation, but the former opioid produced longer postoperative analgesia. [56] Diamorphine 250 μg combined with fentanyl 15 μg as additive to spinal bupivacaine were not superior to diamorphine alone. [57] Sarvan et al [58] found in 200 cesarean done under spinal anaesthesia with 12.5 mg hyperbaric bupivacaine that the ED [95] of 400 μg subarachnoid diamorphine is needed to prevent intraoperative analgesic supplementation. This high dose increased time for first request postoperative analgesic, but also augmented the incidence of nausea, vomiting and pruritus. The addition of intrathecal diamorphine does not appear to influence block height. [60]

Fentanyl. Is the oldest synthetic piperidine opioid agonist, 100 to 80 times more potent than morphine, chemically identified as N-[1-phenethyl-4-piperidyl) propionanilide citrate [1:1] with a molecular weight of 528.60. The empirical formula is $C_{22}H_{28}N_2O \bullet C_6H_8O_7$. The pharmacokinetics of fentanyl can be described as a three-compartment model, with a distribution time of 1.7 minutes, redistribution of 13 minutes and a terminal elimination half-life of 219 minutes. The volume of distribution for fentanyl is 4 L/kg. It is primarily transformed in the liver, demonstrates a high first pass clearance and releases approximately 75% of an intravenous dose in urine, mostly as metabolites with less than 10% representing the unchanged drug. It has a rapid onset of action when the drug is given intravenously or intrathecally. Fentanyl has less emetic activity than either morphine or petidine. [27, 28, 30, 32]

After intrathecal morphine, fentanyl is probably the most widely used opioid in patients undergoing cesarean section; improves quality of spinal anaesthesia, reduces dose of local anaesthetics, but has little impact on prolonging postoperative analgesia. [60, 61, 62] Most used doses of intrathecal fentanyl range from 15 to 25 μg, although this opioid had been investigated in a wide range as of 2.5 up to 50 μg for cesarean delivery. It can be safely mixed with lidocaine, bupivacaine, levobupivacaine, ropivacaine, or mepivacaine. [63, 64, 65, 66] The first study using intrathecal fentanyl was done by Hunt at [67] from Brigham and Women´s Hospital in Boston USA; they evaluated 0, 2.5, 5, 6.25, 12.5, 25, 37.5 and 50 μg of fentanyl added to spinal hyperbaric bupivacaine 0.75% in 56 parturients undergoing cesarean delivery. Sixty seven percent of patients in the control group needed supplemental intraoperative opioids. None of the parturients who received more than 6.5 μg fentanyl required transoperative opioids. Time for first analgesic request was 33.7±30.8 min (mean±SD) in the control group and increased to 130±30 min ($p<0.05$] in those women treated with 6.25 μg fentanyl. Duration of effective analgesia was significantly longer in this group 192±74.9 min versus 71.8±43.2 min ($p<0.05$]. Bigger doses had no effect on effective analgesia. Itching was increased with 25 and 50 μg. There were no side effects in the neonates. They concluded that the optimal dose of spinal fentanyl is 6.5 μg. Most authors reported that higher doses from 12.5 to 25 μg [68, 69] are safe and enhance spinal blockade, trans cesarean analgesia and immediate postsurgical analgesia, without increasing side effects.

The optimal dose of 12 mg 0.5% hyperbaric bupivacaine for C-section was reduced to 8 mg adding 10 μg of spinal fentanyl. [71] The addition of fentanyl 20 μg to 10 mg hyperbaric bupivacaine 0.5% did not alter significantly spirometric parameters in 40 parturients after cesarean delivery compared with bupivacaine alone. [72]

In summary, the addition of intrathecal fentanyl to local anaesthetics used in cesarean section reduces the need for intraoperative analgesics, improves postoperative analgesia for a brief period of time of 2-4 hours, has no effect on the subsequent analgesic doses. The aforementioned doses are very safe for the mother and newborn, and its side effects are minimal.

Sufentanil citrate. Synthesized in mid-1970s, was introduced into clinical practice 10 years later. Sufentanil is a potent pure agonist opioid, 6-10 times more potent than fentanyl, chemically designated as N-{4-(Methoxymethyl)-1-[2-[2-thienyl)ethyl]-4-piperidinyl}-N-phenylpropanamide, with a molecular weight of 578.68. The molecular formula is $C_{22}H_{30}N_2O_2S$. [73, 74]

This opioid is a fundamental part of daily anaesthesia armamentarium. As spinal additive for cesarean section, sufentanil had been used in doses ranging from 1.5 to 20 μg. The initial clinical research by Courtney et al [75] compared 0, 10, 15 and 20 μg as spinal adjuvant to 0.75% hyperbaric bupivacaine 10.5 mg in 37 women undergoing elective cesarean delivery. Analgesia was prolonged significantly in all patients treated with sufentanil, but pruritus incidence was notably increased. Apgar score and Early Neonatal Neurobehavioral Scale were within normal limits. The most recommended dosages range from 2.5 to 5 μg improving spinal anaesthesia and postoperative analgesia, with mild side effects. [28, 76, 77, 78, 79] Braga and coworkers [78] compared sufentanil 0, 2.5, 5 and 7.5 μg added to spinal hyperbaric bupivacaine 12.5 mg. Onset block was significantly shorter in women treated with the opioid and postoperative analgesia was longer in patients receiving 5 and 7.5 μg sufentanil. Those women who received higher doses had more incidences of sedation and pruritus. A prospective, randomized, double-blind, controlled trial [79] found that smaller doses also produced excellent operative analgesia and prolonged postcesarean analgesia; the authors compared 0, 1.5, 2.5 and 5 μg sufentanil added to hyperbaric bupivacaine 0.5% 12.5 mg in 100 pregnant women undergoing elective C-section. Women treated with the opioid had no operative pain, postoperative analgesia was prolonged and rescue analgesic was similar in those women treated with sufentanil. Itch was more frequent in the 2.5 and 5 μg sufentanil groups than in placebo or 1.5 μg sufentanil. There were no differences in the newborn evaluation. Bang et al [80] compared a placebo group versus 2.5 versus 5 μg sufentanil added to spinal hyperbaric bupivacaine and reported no significant differences among the 3 groups regarding the maximum sensory levels and motor block. Patients receiving 5 μg sufentanil had slower recovery of the sensory block. Intrathecal sufentanil enhanced intraoperative analgesia, muscle relaxation and duration of effective analgesia in a dose related response. Occurrence of hypotension, sedation, and itching were also opiate dose related. The addition of 2.5 μg sufentanil to 0.5% levobupivacaine produced faster onset time for sensory and motor block than levobupivacaine alone. It also prolonged postoperative analgesia and reduced analgesic needs. These results were similar to the addition of intrathecal 10 μg fentanyl. [81] Sufentanil 5 μg added to spinal local anaesthetics produce similar results as spinal morphine 200 μg regarding anaesthesia quality, operative analgesia, incidence of maternal emesis as well as newborn safety, but morphine postoperative analgesia was longer 19.5± 4.7 hours versus 6.3±5.2 hours $p< 0.05$]. [28, 82]

Adding 5 μg sufentanil to ropivacaine appears to be optimal, as it increases the efficacy of spinal analgesia without increasing the incidence of side effects, and ropivacaine dose can be reduced up to 28% of ED50 for C-section. [83, 84, 85] Mixing 5 or 10 μg sufentanil with 75 mg lidocaine 5% in parturients undergoing cesarean delivery prolonged spinal anaesthesia compared to placebo, but also produced mild to moderate respiratory depression, which was more important with 10 μg 46.7% ($p<0.001$]. [86]

Several authors had compared fentanyl versus equianalgesic doses of intrathecal sufentanil administered concurrently with hyperbaric bupivacaine 0.5% for cesarean delivery; both opioids abolished intraoperative opioid requirements, and discreetly prolonged postcesarean analgesia although sufentanil produced more prolonged analgesia without significative side effects on the parturient and neonate. [87, 88, 89]. Bremerich et al [90] reported that the association of sufentanil-levobupivacaine was better than fentanyl added to intrathecal bupivacaine o levobupivacaine. A study from Brasil [91] showed that intrathecal sufentanil 2.5 μg combined with morphine 80 μg during anaesthesia with hyperbaric bupivacaine decreased significantly the immediate incidence of postcesarean shivering from 62.5% to 32.5% ($p<0.007$].

*Meperidine (Pethidine).*Meperidine is a synthetic opioid agent, and is the only opioid that has significant local anaesthetic activity in the dose range normally used for analgesia. Was synthesized in 1939 as an anticholinergic agent, but was soon discovered to have analgesic properties. It belongs to the phenylpiperidine family; it is ethyl 1-methyl-4-phenylisonipecotate hydrochloride, readily soluble in water. Molecular formula is $C_{15}H_{21}NO_2$, and has a molecular weight 247.33274. Meperidine is quickly hydrolyzed in the liver to petidinic acid, and is also demethylated to norpetidine, a neurotoxic metabolite. Meperidine metabolites are further conjugated with glucoronic acid and excreted into the urine. [28, 30, 92, 93].

There are reports using intratecal meperidine mixed with local anaesthetics in several clinical settings; in obstetric patients, meperidine has been used as spinal adjuvant, as a single agent for epidural or subarachnoid for labor pain, and also for anaesthesia-analgesia in cesarean delivery. As spinal sole drug for cesarean section, meperidine had been uses with good results. [94, 95, 96]. Cheun and Kim [96] studied 182 parturients undergoing cesarean delivery; they used meperidine 50 mg combined with 10% dextrose 0.5 mL injected in the lumbar spinal space achieving sensory and motor blockade in all patients, prolonged analgesia [453±158.1 min) and motor recovery [75.9±17.2 min). Side effects were minimum and included nausea, hypotension and pruritus. Eighteen patients had mild pain at the end of surgery. There were no side effects on the newborns.

Yu and coworkers [97] compared meperidine 10 mg plus intrathecal 0.5% hyperbaric bupivacaine 10 mg versus hyperbaric bupivacaine alone. They found prolonged postcesarean analgesia (mean 234 min, 95% confidence interval 200-269 min) versus control group (mean 125 min, 95% confidence interval 111-138 min; $p<0.001$]. Woman receiving meperidine had more incidence of intraoperative emesis [11 versus 3; p=0.02]. Reducing meperidine dose to 7.5 mg also produces similar results, enhancing local anaesthetics spinal block and prolonging postcesarean analgesia. [98, 99] Meperidine is a good substitute in patients with allergy to local anaesthetics. [100, 101]

Nalbuphine. Is a synthetic agonist-antagonist opioid belonging to the phenanthrene group. Chemically is 17-(cyclobutylmethy1]-4, 5a-epoxymorphinan-36a, 14-triol hydrochloride, molecular weight 393.91, soluble in water [35.5 mg/mL at 25°C) and ethanol [0.8%), Pka 8.71 and 9.96. The molecular formula is $C_{21}H_{27}NO_4$ HCl. It is structurally related to naloxone, an antagonist of the opiate receptors, and to oxymorphone, an analgesic agonist of the opiate receptors. It has an elimination half-life (t1/20] of about 5 hours in normal people. Because nalbuphine is mainly eliminated from the body by biotransformation, nalbuphine undergoes an extensive first-pass metabolism. [102, 103]

Rawal and coworkers studied several spinal opioids in sheep, including nalbuphine; [104] although spinal nalbuphine was not the less neurotoxic, the authors found that this opioid was associated with relative minor behavioral and EEG changes, sedation, spinal cord mild inflammatory and neuronal changes. Following intrathecal nalbuphine, the above-mentioned changes were similar to those seen in control animals. One animal developed motor impairment during 60 minutes. The analgesic effect of spinal nalbuphine can be reverted by naloxone. [105] To date, no clinical reports of this opioid have mentioned secondary neurological damage, although this observation has not enough clinical evidence. There is little clinical research with this opioid injected intrathecally. Nalbuphine been used as additive for spinal anaesthesia in several clinical settings in doses from 200 to 1600 μg. [106, 107, 108]

The first study with intrathecal nalbuphine in obstetric patients was conducted by Culebras et al; [109] in a double blind study they injected nalbuphine 200, 800, 1600 μg mixed with hyperbaric 0.5% bupivacaine versus morphine 200 μg with bupivacaine in 90 parturients undergoing cesarean delivery. Only women receiving morphine and nalbuphine 200 μg reported transoperative pain. In the nalbuphine groups, postoperative analgesia lasted longest with the 0.8 mg dose, but postoperative analgesia was significantly prolonged in the morphine group (p<0.0001]. Itching incidence was superior with spinal morphine as well as postcesarean nausea and vomiting. There was no maternal or newborn respiratory depression. Culebra´s article was accompanied by an editorial written by Yaksh; [110] most of his commentaries were regarding the lack of solid evidence about the neurotoxicity of nalbuphine and emphasized that benefits does not outweigh the risks to use this the opioid by the spinal route.

Yoon et al [111] found that an intrathecal mixture of nalbuphine 1000 μg, morphine 100 μg and hyperbaric 0.5% bupivacaine 10 mg for cesarean delivery strengthen intraoperative analgesia compared with morphine alone, but this combination reduce postcesarean duration of complete analgesia and had no effect on the incidence of itch. In a recent randomized, double blind article using intrathecal nalbuphine for postcaesarean analgesia there were no differences between nalbuphine 800 μg versus 25 μg fentanyl associated with hyperbaric 0.5% bupivacaine 10 mg; both opioids produce transoperative analgesia and early postoperative analgesia. [112]

4. Spinal opioids side effects

As described in the preceding paragraphs, intrathecal opioids as adjuncts to local anaesthetics are very safe in spinal anaesthesia for cesarean section, although may have sporadic potentially life-threatening events. There is variety of side effects which are worth to be discussed briefly. These side effects are due to different factors such as pharmacological and pharmacodynamic characteristics of each opioid, the injected dose, and type of patient. Opioids with high liposolubility have less risk of rostral migration and lower incidence of CNS side effects. Larger doses will have higher incidence and severity of CNS deleterious effects.

Respiratory depression is a deleterious side effect which may have serious consequences like respiratory arrest and even death. Fortunately, it is a very rare event. This complication can occurs as quickly as 15 to 20 minutes after injection of lipophilic opioids, but with water soluble opioids the event is late. [113, 114, 115] Morphine intrathecal doses higher than 300 μg are associated with more episodes of respiratory depression. [116] It is mandatory to closely monitor all patients receiving neuroaxial opioids. Besides clinical surveillance, pulse oximetry monitors are used by most clinicians, although the use of transcutaneous carbon dioxide monitor has been recommended recently. [117] It is prudent to give prophylactic nasal oxygen. When respiratory depression is detected, it should be managed with intravenous naloxone. Also intravenous nalbuphine has been used with excellent results. On rare occasions it is necessary to use ventilatory support with endotracheal intubation.

Emesis and pruritus are the most frequent side effects. Nausea and vomiting are similar, but pruritus increased in direct proportion to the dose of intrathecal morphine (linear regression, p=0.0001]. Although emesis due to spinal morphine do not interfere with early feeding after surgical delivery, [118] it is an unpleasant nuisance that can be prevented by various drugs administered immediately after the umbilical cord is ligated; ondansetron 4-8 mg, ganisetron 3 mg, tropisetron 5, droperidol 1.25 mg, dexamethasone 4-8 mg and diphenydramine 30 mg. [119, 120] Metoclopramide 10 mg does not appear to be effective for emesis prophylaxis in this patient population. Serotonin [5-HT3] receptors antagonists had poor effect preventing itching, while the prophylactic or therapeutic administration of droperidol 1.25. mg, nalbuphine 5-10 mg, pèntazocine 15 mg, butorphanol 1 mg followed by intravenous infusion of 0.2 mg/h. [121, 122, 123]

Severe postoperative hypothermia has been described in a variety of surgical procedures, including cesarean section done under epidural or spinal therapeutic doses of morphine. The mechanism is not well known but it is said that could be mediated by morphine cephalad spinal spread reaching opioid receptors and altering the temperature set point in the hypothalamus. It can be treated effectively with naloxone or lorazepam. [124-129]

5. Non opioids spinal additives

As we reviewed, spinal opioids side effect profiles may have some limitation to be used as adjuvants in cesarean delivery; pruritus, nausea, vomiting, and urinary retention are non fatal deleterious side effects but bother most patients. Late respiratory arrest and hypothermia after usual opioid doses has been seldom reported in the literature. There are several non-opioide adjuvants that have been studied for the purpose to enhance spinal anaesthesia and to prolong and augment postcesarean analgesia [130], being alpha2 agonists the most promising agents. [131, 132] Spinal adjuvants like magnesium, ketamine, neostigmine are mostly used for clinical research, and nowadays is no prudent to recommend these drugs as a routine practice. *Clonidine.* Eisenach et al demonstrated that epidural/spinal clonidine did not affect sheep fetus, but fetal bradycardia may limit the efficacy of spinal clonidine if used more than 10 μg/kg in obstetrics. [133, 134] Many clinical studies have been done using neuroaxial clonidine mixed with local anaesthetics and/or opioids, and as solo drug in obstetrics patients. Low doses of spinal clonidine in subarachnoid anaesthesia for cesarean delivery are reported to enhance the anaesthetic block, to reduce dose of local anaesthetics, and to extend postoperative analgesia. There are studies mixing clonidine with intrathecal opioids, as there is a synergic effect.

In a double blind study Filos et al [135] carried out their investigation to evaluate the analgesic effect of sole clonidine in women undergoing elective cesarean delivery, 150 μg were injected 45 minutes after general anaesthesia and compared to intrathecal saline as control group. Pain intensity was lower in clonidine treated parturients 20 to 120 minutes after spinal injection ($p<0.05$], request for first analgesic was also longer in the clonidine group 414±128 minutes versus 181±169 minutes ($p<0.01$]. Clonidine side effects were severe; hypotension with a maximal reduction of systolic [15±9%), diastolic [22±12%) and mean arterial pressure [18±12%). Sedation was significantly more intense compared to saline ($p<0.05$]; also dried mouth was more commonly ($p<0.01$]. Although these data suggest that 150 μg subarachnoid clonidine is effective to treat acute pain after cesarean section, it has side effects such as hypotension, sedation, and dryness of mouth. Two years later, the same authors [136] performed a different study comparing 150, 350 and 450 μg of spinal clonidine to evaluate the dose-response hemodynamic and analgesic responses in the immediate postoperative period of cesarean section under general anaesthesia. They found less pain in all groups in a dose dependent mode: request for first analgesic 402±75 min, 570±76 min, and 864±80 minutes respectively ($p<0.01$-0.001]. Clonidine reduced mean arterial pressure compared with baseline only in those patients treated with 150 μg [21±13%, $p<0.05$]. Sedation was evident in all groups. Respiratory rate and motor activity of the lower extremities were unaffected in all three groups. The hemodynamic stability after 300 and 450 μg suggested a pressor consequence at peripheral sites. This investigation demonstrated a dose related analgesia after spinal clonidine at doses as great as 450 μg. Studies with lower doses of clonidine has shown satisfactory results. Peach et al [137] in a randomized, double blind trial compared intrathecal clonidine mixed with fentanyl 15 μg and morphine μg versus clonidine plus morphine in 240 women undergoing cesarean delivery with hyperbaric 0.5% bupivacaine. Using a dose finding analysis the authors found similar comparable postoperative efficacy and side effects for groups receiving morphine 100 μg with clonidine 60, 90, or 150 μg and concluded that a multimodal approach for postcesarean analgesia, using subarachnoid bupivacaine, fentanyl, morphine 100 μg, and clonidine 60 μg, improves pain relief compared with morphine 100 μg or clonidine 150 μg alone, but increases intraoperative sedation and may increase perioperative vomiting. Other investigators have found that clonidine 75 μg is a safe dose; prolong the anesthetic block and enhance postoperative analgesia, with minimal side effects and no harm to the newborn [132, 138, 139] Van Tuijl et al [140] compared 15 μg, 30 μg and 60 μg of clonidine added to hyperbaric bupivacaine 0.5%; the authors found a dose dependent variability of analgesia duration and sedation. Duration of analgesia was significantly higher in those patients who received clonidine 60 μg as compared to the other two groups [598.7±140.47 versus 436.65±149.84 and 387.1±97.05 min respectively). Sedation was also more in the highest dose. In this study the authors recommended 15 μg and 30 μg doses due to good postoperative analgesia and less sedation.

It has been mentioned that mixture of hyperbaric local anaesthetics with clonidine should not be done in one syringe before injection into the subarachnoid space, but to inject each drug in separate syringes in order to avoid syringe interactions, in particular changes in the density of local anaesthetics. Sachan et al [141] studied the differences between hyperbaric bupivacaine mixed with clonidine in the same syringe just prior to subarachnoid injection versus separate administration in 60 parturient undergoing cesarean deliveries. Those women who received clonidine 75 μg plus hyperbaric bupivacaine 0.5% 10 mg contained in one syringe had shorter analgesia time [337±18.22 min) versus those patients receiving same drugs but applied in separated syringes [474.33±20.79 min), p=0.000. Moreover, time to reach highest sensory level and complete motor block was significantly less, without any major haemodynamic instability in those women injected in a sequentially manner. As a single drug, subarachnoid clonidine is not recommended for anaesthesia neither for postcaesarean analgesia.

Should we administer intrathecal clonidine in obstetric patients? Under the results of clinical investigations done by many authors in different countries, intrathecal clonidine is a safe drug in obstetric patients when recommended doses are observed, but more clinical studies are needed to adequately respond to this question. [131] Moreover, we have to keep in mind that the FDA maintains its recommendation not to use epidural clonidine in obstetrics. This organization does not mention the use of intrathecal clonidine in this clinical scenario. For more information about intrathecal clonidine please read the chapter entitled *Intrathecal clonidine as spinal anaesthesia adjuvant. Is there a magical dose?* included in this book.

Midazolam. A water soluble imidazobenzodiazepine, highly liposoluble in vivo, with a rapid onset of action and high metabolic clearance. Chemically is 8-chloro-6-[2-fluorophenyl)-1-methyl-4*H*-imidazo [1, 5-a] [1, 4] benzodiazepine hydrochloride, and the molecular formula $C_{18}H_{13}ClFN_3 \bullet HCl$, with a molecular weight of 362.25. [142] For an extended information on midazolam, we refer you to the chapter included in this book entitled *Midazolam in spinal anaesthesia: intrathecal or intravenous?* written by Beyazit Zencirci.

A preservative free midazolam administered by continuous intrathecal infusion to sheep and pigs in doses from 5 to 15 mg/day during 43 days demonstrated that behavior, neurological function, and vital signs were normal. There were no data of neurological damage, except mild inflammation surrounding the catheter tract that was also observed in animals treated with placebo. [143] There are few articles using intrathecal midazolam for cesarean section. In a prospective, randomized, double-blind, placebo controlled study [144] the authors compared

1 and 2 mg of midazolam added to subarachnoid bupivacaine 10 mg versus plain bupivacaine. Request for first analgesic was 4.3±0.7 versus 6.1±1.0 versus 3.8±0.5 hours, respectively. Supplemental diclofenac were significantly less in those women treated with midazolam 2 mg [93±29 mg) compared with midazolam 1 mg [148±16 mg) and plain bupivacaine [145±12 mg). Time to block regression was longer in plain bupivacaine group B [182±30 minutes) compared with midazolam 1 mg [152±32 minutes) and midazolam 2 mg group B [126±20 minutes) (both p<.001]. Interesting, patient who did not receive intrathecal midazolam had higher incidence of nausea and vomiting. Arterial pressure, heart rate, oxygen saturation, sedation score, and time to first void were comparable between groups. Karbasfrushan et al [145]. compared intrathecal midazolam 2 mg added to bupivacaine 10 mg versus plain bupivacaine in women undergoing elective cesarean. Patients treated with midazolam had significant pain relieve at 15 and 120 min after surgery, but there were no significant differences between the groups regarding the intensity of pain 5, 30, 60 and 240 min after the surgery. Request for first analgesic was 178.06±77.33 versus 142.18±55.19 min. Duration of analgesia and regression for sensory analgesia was similar in both groups, but nausea and vomiting were higher in the midazolam group. Salimi et al [147] use a combination of 2 mg midazolam plus 5 µg sufentanyl intrathecally versus sufentanyl alone for labour pain in 80 parturients. Analgesia was enhanced and prolonged significantly [185±15.2 min versus 92±12.7 min p=0.001]. No significant side effects were observed in both groups.

Magnesium sulfate. Is a chemical compound containing magnesium, sulfur and oxygen. Magnesium sulphate is a noncompetitive antagonist of the N-methyl-d-aspartate (NMDA) receptor, therefore can interfere nociceptive modulation. There is controversy about the neurotoxicity of magnesium sulfate injected into the neuraxis. [148, 149] In a contemporary study conducted in Sprague-Dawley rats, Ozdogan and coworkers [149] were able to demonstrate on electron microscopic examinations, that single or repeated spinal injection of magnesium sulphate 0.15% produced significant neurodegeneration. Nonetheless, there are clinical studies that support the use of this ion via neuraxial-epidural or subarachnoid-in diverse clinical scenarios, [150, 151, 152] including in the obstetric field, showing to prolong analgesia without important side effects in healthy and pathologic parturients.

It has been used through epidural [153, 154] and spinal via for cesarean delivery, with highly variable results. Ghrab et al [155] studied 105 women undergoing cesarean section with spinal anaesthesia. They found that adding magnesium sulphate 100 mg to morphine 100 µg improved the quality and duration of postcesarean analgesia without augmenting the incidence of harmful side effects. Jabalameli and Pakzadmoghadam [156] compared 0, 50, 75 and 100 mg magnesium sulphate added to spinal bupivacaine in 132 parturients undergoing cesarean delivery. Magnesium produced a delay in the onset of sensory and motor blockade. Duration of sensory and motor blockade were longer in those women treated with 75 a 100 mg doses. Patients who did not receive magnesium had a shorter recovery time and needed more postoperative analgesic (p<0.001]. In patients with mild preeclampsia [157] adding magnesium sulphate 50 mg to 0.5% hyperbaric bupivacaine and fentanyl 25 µg induced a slower onset of motor and sensory block, prolonged duration of spinal anaesthesia and motor block and reduced needs of diclofenac during 24 hours. No harmful side effects were noticed. As Faiz et al mentioned, spinal magnesium improved perioperative shivering in women undergoing elective caesarean delivery. [158] In a prospective, randomized, double blind study in 90 women undergoing cesarean section, Unlugenc et al [159] were unable to probe that 50 mg magnesium sulphate have any benefit over spinal anaesthesia with bupivacaine 0.5%. Adding this adjuvant to 10 mg spinal bupivacaine did not shorten onset time of sensory and motor blockade or prolonged duration of subarachnoid anaesthesia as compared to spinal fentanyl.

6. Conclusions

Across the world, subarachnoid anaesthesia is the most used anaesthetic procedure for Cesarean delivery. Compared to general and epidural anaesthesia, its main disadvantage is a short duration action and most important, the lack of prolonged postoperative analgesia. These two negative factors had been overcome with the addition of drugs that act enhancing quality and durability, while they managed to decrease the dose of local anaesthetic and prolong postoperative analgesia. Provision of postcesarean delivery analgesia is of great consequence since it accelerate early ambulation, decreases maternal morbidity, improves parturient outcome, decrease cost, and most important augment the quality of the mother-infant relationship from the moment of birth.

When planning spinal anaesthesia for cesarean section there are different local anaesthetics and various adjuvants that enhance the technique and favor better outcome of our patients. It is vital that the choice of adjuvants drugs be rationally and according to each clinical condition and local availability of these drugs. Although there is no gold standard for a perfect spinal anaesthesia and postcesarean analgesia, in this millennium is mandatory to provide the best available care. As reviewed, there is a large list of options and the choice is mostly determined by drug safety and accessibility, the experience of anaesthesiologists, and monetary factors.

When adjuvants are selected for neuroaxial anaesthesia, it is mandatory to use drugs that are not neurotoxic and are free of preservatives.

Spinal Adjuvants	Dose range in µg	Effects	Side effects
Morphine 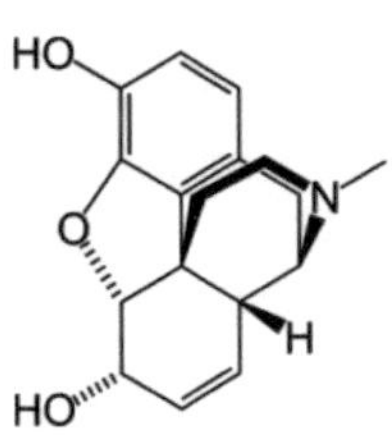	50-400 Recommended dose 100	Reduce DE_{50} and DE_{95} of spinal LA Prolonged POA Reduce analgesics	PONV dose related Pruritus moderate to severe Urinary retention Respiratory depression (rare) Hypothermia (very rare)

http://dx.doi.org/10.5772/58851

Spinal Adjuvants	Dose range in μg	Effects	Side effects
Hydromorphone 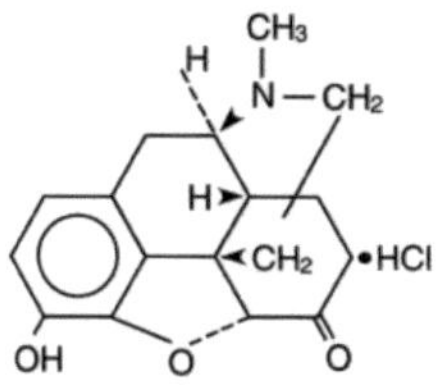	40-100	Prolonged POA Reduce POP analgesics doses	PONV similar no morphine Less itching than morphine
Diamorphine (Heroine) 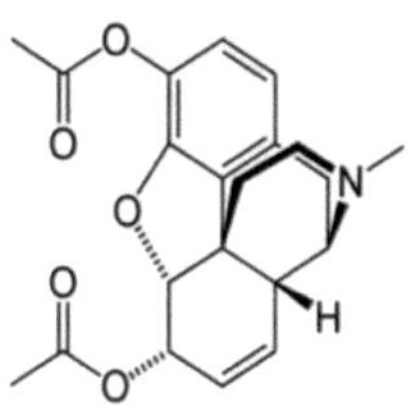	125-400 Recommended dose 300	Reduce intraoperative analgesics Enhance POA Reduce POP analgesics doses	PONV similar no morphine Less itching than morphine
Fentanyl 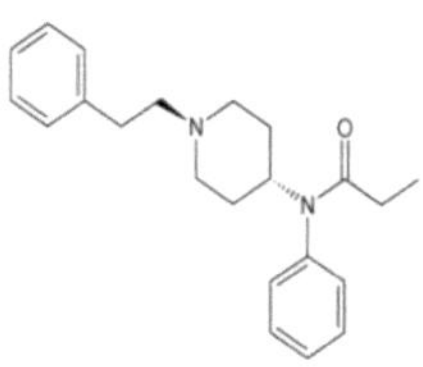	6.5 - 50 Recommended dose 12.5	Fast onset Enhace spinal anaesthesia Reduce spinal LA dose Reduce intraoperative analgesics Enhance POA for 2-4 hours	Less PONV than morphine Less itchichin tha morphine
Sufentanyl 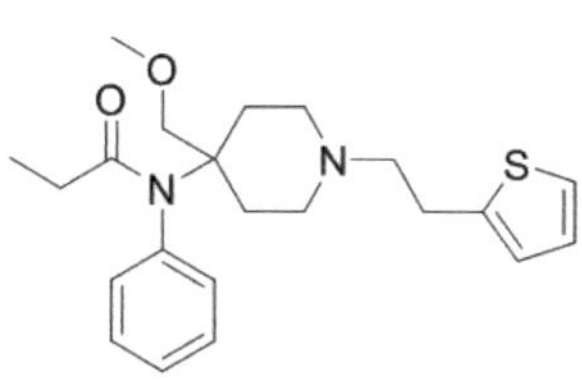	1.5 - 20 Recommended dose 5	Rapid onset Enhace spinal blockade Reduce spinal LA doses Improve trans cesarean analgesia Short prolongation of POA Reduce PO analgesic needs	Dose relates itchnig Posoperative sedation PONV higher than fentanyl
Meperidine 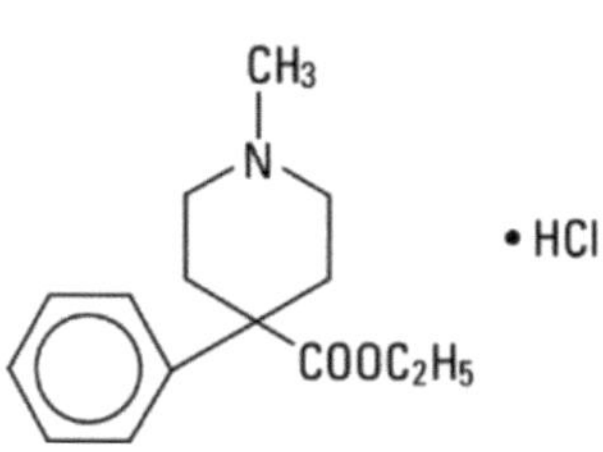	7000 to 10, 000 D Recommended dose, 500	Rapid onset Improve spinal anaesthesia Prolongs POA	High incidence of transurgical vomitig PONV are high

Spinal Adjuvants	Dose range in µg	Effects	Side effects
Nalbufine* 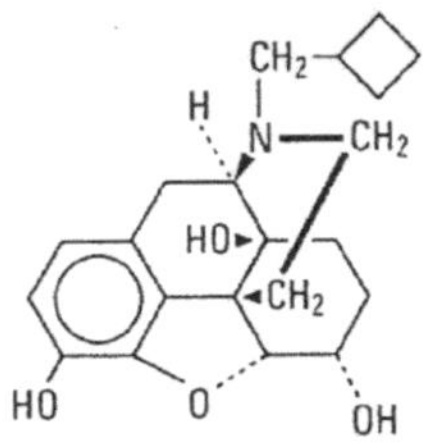 • HCl	200 - 1600 Recommended dose 800	Enhance operative analgesia Prolongs arly POA No effect on itching	PONV are dose related In not better that spinal morphine
Clonidine 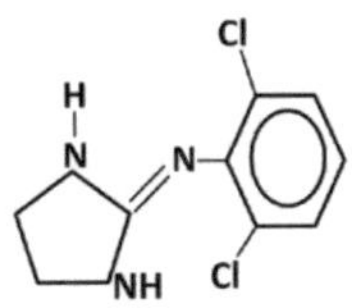 • HCl	15 - 450 Recommended dose 30	Improve spinal anaesthesia Reduce spinal LA dose Prolongs POA No respiratory depresion	Hypothension Sedation Dry mouth Fetal and maternal bradycardia
Midazolam* 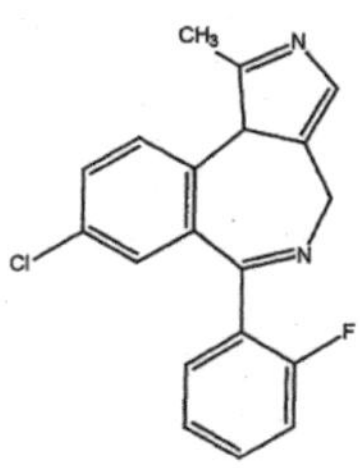 (I),	1000-2000 Recommended dose 2000?	Enhance POA Reduce PO analgesic doses Reduce PONV?	Augments PONV?
Magnesium sulphate* 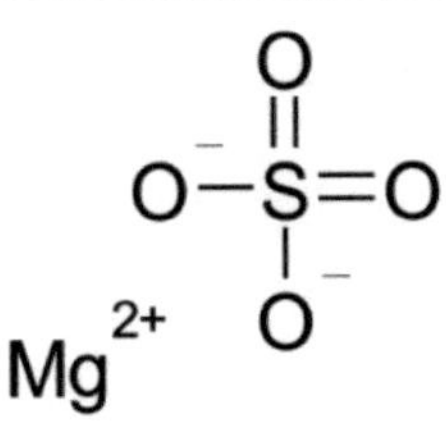	5, 000-100, 000 Recommended dose?	Prolongs spinal block Augments POA Reduces PO analgesic doses Reduces postoperative shivering	Delays onset of spinal anaesthesia

LA=Local anaesthetics. POA=Postoperative analgesia. POP=Postoperative. PONV=Postoeprative nausea and vomiting.

*Nalbuphine, midazolam and magnesium suphate are under clinical investigatior to determine its use in spinal anaesthesia for several clinical scenarios.

Table 1. Spinal additives and some drugs under clinical research in parturients undergoing cesarean delivery with spinal anaesthesia.

Acknowledgements

First of all, I dedicate this chapter to my Great Allah, my parents, and to my son Ahmed, my lovely daughter Yasmine.

I also thank Dr Juan C. Flores-Carrillo and Dr Víctor Whizar-Lugo for their help and patient.

I hope this chapter help reader and add some helpful information.

Author details

Hala M. Goma[1*], Juan C. Flores-Carrillo[2] and Víctor Whizar-Lugo[3]

*Address all correspondence to: ahmeda1995@yahoo.com

1 Faculty of Medicine, Cairo University, Egypt

2 Anaesthesia and Critical Care, Instituto Mexicano del Seguro Social, Tijuana, México

3 Anaesthesia, Critical Care and Pain Medicine, Hospital General de Tijuana, ISESALUD, Tijuana, México

References

[1] D´Angelo R, Smiley RM, Riley, Segal S. The serious complication repository project of the Society for Obstetric Anesthesia and Perinatology. Anesyhesiology 2014;120:1505-12.

[2] Simkin P. Moving beyond the debate: a holistic approach to understanding and treating effects of neuraxial analgesia. Birth. 2012;39:327-32.

[3] Butwick A. What's new in obstetric anesthesia in 2011? Reducing maternal adverse outcomes and improving obstetric anesthesia quality of care. Anesth Analg. 2012;115:1137-45.

[4] Whizar LV, Carrillo FC, Puerta RG. Complicaciones neurológicas de la anestesia neuroaxial. In: Anestesia obstétrica. Canto SAL, Higgins GLF, editors. Anestesia obstétrica. Segunda edición. México DF. Manual Moderno. 2008. p. 379-397.

[5] Dharmalingam TK, Ahmad Zainuddin NA. Survey on maternal satisfaction in receiving spinal anaesthesia for caesarean section. Malays J Med Sci. 2013;20:51-4.

[6] Aiono-Le TL, Butwick AJ, Carvalho B. A survey of perioperative anesthetics practices for cesarean delivery. Anesthesiol Res Pract. 2009;Article ID 5106442.

[7] Butterworth J. Physiology of spinal anesthesia: what are the implications for management? Reg Anesth Pain Med. 1998;23:370-3.

[8] Roofthooft E, Van de Velde M. Low-dose spinal anaesthesia for caesarean section to prevent spinal-induced hypotension. Curr Opin Anaesthesiol. 2008;21:259-62.

[9] Rodgers A, Walker N and Schug S. Reduction of postoperative mortality and morbidity with epidural or spinal anesthesia. Results from overview of randomized trials. Brit Med J 2000; 321:1493.

[10] El-Gilany AH, Abdel-Hady DM. Newborn first feed and prelacteal feeds in Mansoura, Egypt. Biomed Res Int. 2014;2014:258470.

[11] Khanal V, Adhikari M, Sauer K, Zhao Y. Factors associated with the introduction of prelacteal feeds in Nepal: findings from the Nepal demographic and health survey 2011. Int Breastfeed J. 2013;8:9.

[12] Marín Gabriel MÁ, del Rey Hurtado de Mendoza B, Jiménez Figueroa L, et al. Analgesia with breastfeeding in addition to skin-to-skin contact during heel prick. Arch Dis Child Fetal Neonatal Ed. 2013;98:F499-503.

[13] Imarengiaye CO, Akhideno I, Omoifo EC. Characteristics of postpartum pain associated with vaginal and caesarean births. West Afr J Med. 2014;33:3-6.

[14] Landau R, Bollag L, Ortner C. Chronic pain after childbirth. Int J Obstet Anesth. 2013:22:133-45.

[15] Matsuki A. Nothing new under the sun-A Japanese pioneer in the clinical use of intrathecal morphine. Anesthesiology 1983;58:289-90.

[16] Pert CB, Snyder SH. Opiate receptor: demonstration in nervous tissue. Science 1973;179:1011-14.

[17] Yaksh TL, Rudy TA. Analgesia mediated by a direct spinal action of narcotics. Science 1976;192:1357-1358.

[18] Hindle A. Intrathecal opioids in the management of acute postoperative pain. Contin Educ Anaesth Crit Care Pain. 2008;8:81-5.

[19] Jaffe RA, Rowe MA. A comparison of the local anesthetic effects of meperidine, fentanyl, and sufentanil on dorsal root axons. Anesth Analg. 1996;83:776-81.

[20] Kerchner GA, Zhuo M. Presynaptic suppression of dorsal horn inhibitory transmission by mu-opioid receptors. J Neurophysiol. 2002;88:520-2.

[21] Bujedo BM, Santos SG, Azpiazu AU. A review of epidural and intrathecal opioids used in the management of postoperative pain. J Opioid Manag. 2012;8:177-92.

[22] Bujedo BM. Spinal opioid bioavailability in postoperative pain. Pain Pract. 2014;14:350-64.

[23] Rawal N, Nuutinen L, Raj PP, et al. Behavioral and histopathologic effects following intrathecal administration of butorphanol, sufentanil, and nalbuphine in sheep. Anesthesiology 1991;75:1025-34.

[24] Alici HA, Ozmen I, Cesur M, Sahin F. Effect of the spinal drug tramadol on the fatty acid compositions of rabbit spinal cord and brain. Biol Pharm Bull. 2003;26:1403-6.

[25] Ozmen I, Naziroğlu M, Alici HA, et al. Spinal morphine administration reduces the fatty acid contents in spinal cord and brain by increasing oxidative stress. Neurochem Res. 2007;32:19-25.

[26] Yaksh TL, Allen JW, Veesart SL, et al. Role of meningeal mast cells in intrathecal morphine-evoked granuloma fromation. Anesthesiology 2013;118:664-78

[27] De Gregori S, De Gregori M, Ranzani GN, et al.Morphine metabolism, transport and brain disposition. Metab Brain Dis. 2012;27:1-5.

[28] Trescot A, Datta S, Lee M, Hansen H. Opioid pharmacology. Pain Physician 2008;11:S133-53.

[29] Orbach-Zinger S, Ioscovich A, Aviram A, et al. National survey of postoperative pain control after cesarean delivery. Isr Med Assoc J. 2014;16:153-6.

[30] Tsen LC. Anesthesia for cesarean delivery. In: Chestnut D, Wong C, Ysen LC, Ngan W, Beilin G, Mhyre J. editors. Chestnut´s Obstetrics anesthesia: Principles and practice. Fifth edition. Philadelphia. Elsevier-Saunders. 2014. p. 545-603.

[31] Sullivan JT. Neuroaxial blockade for obstetric surgery. In: Wong AC. editor. Spinal and epidural anesthesia. New York. McGraw Hill. 2007. p. 281-304.

[32] Canto SL. Opioides neuroaxiales en anestesia obstétrica. In: Anestesia obstétrica. Canto SAL, Higgins GLF. editors. Anestesia obstétrica. Segunda edición. México DF. Manual Moderno. 2008. p. 67-73.

[33] Girgin NK, Gurbet A, Turker G, Aksu H, Gulhan N. Intrathecal morphine in anesthesia for cesarean delivery: dose-response relationship for combinations of low-dose intrathecal morphine and spinal bupivacaine. J Clin Anesth. 2008;20:180-5.

[34] Karaman S, Kocabas S, Uyar M, Hayzaran S, Firat V. The effects of sufentanil or morphine added to hyperbaric bupivacaine in spinal anaesthesia for caesarean section. Eur J Anaesthesiol. 2006;23:285-91.

[35] Dualé C, Frey C, Bolandard F, Barrière A, Schoeffler P. Epidural versus intrathecal morphine for postoperative analgesia after caesarean section. Br J Anaesth. 2003;91:690-4.

[36] Cortes BB, Segura LF, Alba VH. Analgesia postcesárea con morfina intratecal: 100 μg versus 200 μg. Anest Mex. 2005;17:122-16.

[37] Villalba RS, García SJ, García HJ. Analgesia postoperatoria con morfina subaracnoidea en cesárea electiva. Rev Sanid Milit Mex. 2007;61: 86-90.

[38] Weigl W, Bieryło A, Krzemień-Wiczyńska S, Mayzner-Zawadzka E. Comparative study of postoperative analgesia after intrathecal administration of bupivacaine with fentanyl or morphine for elective caesarean section. Anestezjol Intens Ter. 2009;41:28-32.

[39] Bejar J, Santiago RG, Enrique D. Estudio comparativo de morfina intratecal vs morfina sistémica para analgesia postoperatoria en cesárea. Hospital Universitario de Maternidad y Neonatología. Actas Peru Anestesiol. 2013;21:18-26.

[40] de Carvalo FAC, Tenório SB. Estudio comparativo entre dosis de morfina intratecal para analgesia después de la cesárea. Rev Bras Anestesiol. 2013;63:492-9

[41] Draisci G, Frassanito L, Pinto R, ET AL. Safety and effectiveness of coadministration of intrathecal sufentanil and morphine in hyperbaric bupivacaine-based spinal anesthesia for cesarean section. J Opioid Manag. 2009;5:197-202.

[42] Bouvet L, Da-Col X, Chassard D, et al. ED_{50} and ED_{95} of intrathecal levobupivacaine with opioids for Caesarean delivery. Br J Anaesth. 2011;106:215-20.

[43] Wong JY, Carvalho B, Riley ET. Intrathecal morphine 100 and 200 μg for post-cesarean delivery analgesia: a trade-off between analgesic efficacy and side effects. Int J Obstet Anesth. 2013;22:36-41.

[44] Kanazi GE, Aouad MT, Abdallah FW, et al. The analgesic efficacy of subarachnoid morphine in comparison with ultrasound-guided transversus abdominis plane block after cesarean delivery: a randomized controlled trial. Anesth Analg. 2010;111:475-81.

[45] Loane H, Preston R, Douglas MJ, et al. A randomized controlled trial comparing intrathecal morphine with transversus abdominis plane block for post-cesarean delivery analgesia. Int J Obstet Anesth. 2012;21:112-8.

[46] Murray A, Hagen NA. Hydromorphone. J Pain Symptom Manage. 2005;29(5 Suppl):S57-66.

[47] Rauch E. Intrathecal hydromorphone for postoperative analgesia after cesarean delivery: a retrospective study. AANA J. 2012;80:S25-32.

[48] Beatty NC, Arendt KW, Niesen AD, Wittwer ED, Jacob AK. Analgesia after cesarean delivery: a retrospective comparison of intrathecal hydromorphone and morphine. J Clin Anesth. 2013;25:379-83.

[49] Lee YS, Park YC, Kim JH, et al. Intrathecal hydromorphone added to hyperbaric bupivacaine for postoperative pain relief after knee arthroscopic surgery: a prospective, randomized, controlled trial. Eur J Anaesthesiol. 2012;29:17-21.

[50] Rauch E. Intrathecal hydromorphone for cesarean delivery: in search of improved postoperative pain management: a case report. AANA J. 2011;79:427-32.

[51] Hosztafi S. Heroin, part III: the pharmacology of heroin. Acta Pharm Hung. 2003;73:197-205

[52] Hallworth SP, Fernando R, Bell R, Parry MG, Lim GH. Comparison of intrathecal and epidural diamorphine for elective caesarean section using a combined spinal-epidural technique. Br J Anaesth 1999;82:228-32.

[53] Husaini SW, Russell IF. Intrathecal diamorphine compared with morphine for post-operative analgesia after caesarean section under spinal anaesthesia. Br J Anaesth 1998;81:135-9.

[54] Kelly MC, Carabine UA, Mirakhur RK. Intrathecal diamorphine for analgesia after caesarean section. A dose finding study and assessment of side-effects. Anaesthesia 1998;53:231-7.

[55] Wrench IJ, Sanghera S, Pinder A, Power L, Adams MG. Dose response to intrathecal diamorphine for elective caesarean section and compliance with a national audit standard. Int J Obstet Anesth. 2007;16:17-21.

[56] Cowan CM, Kendall JB, Barclay PM, Wilkes RG. Comparison of intrathecal fentanyl and diamorphine in addition to bupivacaine for caesarean section under spinal anaesthesia. Br J Anaesth. 2002;89:452-8.

[57] Lane S, Evans P, Arfeen Z, Misra U. A comparison of intrathecal fentanyl and diamorphine as adjuncts in spinal anaesthesia for caesarean section. Anaesthesia 2005;60:453-7.

[58] Saravanan S, Robinson AP, Qayoum Dar A, Columb MO, Lyons GR. Minimum dose of intrathecal diamorphine required to prevent intraoperative supplementation of spinal anaesthesia for caesarean section. Br J Anaesth. 2003;91:368-72.

[59] Akerman N, Saxena S, Wilson R, Columb M, Lyons G. Effect of intrathecal diamorphine on block height during spinal anaesthesia for caesarean section with bupivacaine. Br J Anaesth. 2005;94:843.

[60] Biswas BN, Rudra A, Bose BK, et al. Intrathecal fentanyl with hyperbaric bupivacaine improves analgesia during caesarean delivery and in early post-operative period. Indian J Anesth 2002;46:469-72.

[61] Bogra J, Arora N, Srivastava P. Synergistic effect of intrathecal fentanyl and bupivacaine in spinal anesthesia for cesarean section. BMC Anesthesiol. 2005;5:5.

[62] Carvalho B, Butwick A. Postoperative analgesia: Epidural and spinal techniques. In: Chestnut D, Wong C, Ysen LC, Ngan W, Beilin G, Mhyre J. editors. Chestnut's Obstetrics anesthesia: Principles and practice. Fifth edition. Philadelphia. Elsevier-Saunders. 2014. p. 621-661.

[63] Palmer CM, Voulgaropoulos D, Alves D. Subarachnoid fentanyl augments lidocaine spinal anesthesia for cesarean delivery. Reg Anesth. 1995;20:389-94.

[64] Chung CJ, Yun SH, Hwang GB, Park JS, Chin YJ. Intrathecal fentanyl added to hyperbaric ropivacaine for cesarean delivery. Reg Anesth Pain Med. 2002;27:600-3.

[65] Obara M, Sawamura S, Satoh Y, et al. The effect of intrathecal fentanyl added to hyperbaric bupivacaine for caesarean section. Masui 2003;52:378-82.

[66] Bernat GJ, Gallego GJ, Abengochea CA. Estudio aleatorio, doble ciego sobre la utilización de diferentes dosis de bupivacaína hiperbara con o sin fentanilo, en cesáreas con anestesia subaracnoidea. Rev Esp Anestesiol Reanim 2007;54:4-10.

[67] Hunt CO, Naulty JS, Bader AM, et al. Perioperative analgesia with subarachnoid fentanyl-bupivacaine for cesarean delivery. Anesthesiology 1989;71:535-40.

[68] Bano F, Sabbar S, Zafar S, et al. Intrathecal fentanyl as adjunct to hyperbaric bupivacaine in spinal anesthesia for caesarean section. J Coll Physicians Surg Pak. 2006;16:87-90.

[69] Idowu OA, Sanusi AA, Eyelade OR. Effects of intrathecally administered fentanyl on duration of analgesia in patients undergoing spinal anaesthesia for elective caesarean section. Afr J Med Med Sci. 2011;40:213-9.

[70] Meléndez FH. Gamarra HG, Fernández C, Dulcey R. Eficacia del fentanyl adicionado a bupivacaína en el dolor intraoperatorio en cesárea bajo anestesia subaracnoidea. Ensayo clínico controlado. Rev Col Anest. 2005;33:161-63.

[71] Choi DH, Ahn HJ, Kim MH. Bupivacaine-sparing effect of fentanyl in spinal anesthesia for cesarean delivery. Reg Anesth Pain Med. 2000;25:240-5.

[72] Arai YC, Ogata J, Fukunaga K, et al. The effect of intrathecal fentanyl added to hyperbaric bupivacaine on maternal respiratory function during cesarean section. Acta Anaesthesiol Scand. 2006;50:364-7.

[73] Maciejewski D. Sufentanil in anaesthesiology and intensive therapy. Anaesthesiol Int Ther. 2012;44:35-41.

[74] Rosow CE. Sufentanil citrate: a new opioid analgesic for use in anesthesia. Pharmacotherapy 1984;4:11-19.

[75] Courtney MA, Bader AM, Hartwell B, et al. Perioperative analgesia with subarachnoid sufentanil administration. Reg Anesth. 1992;17:274-8.

[76] Vyas N, Sahu DK, Parampill R. Comparative study of intrathecal sufentanil bupivacaine versus intrathecal bupivacaine in patients undergoing elective cesarean section. J Anaesthesiol Clin Pharmacol. 2010 ;26:488-92.

[77] Wang LZ, Zhang YF, Tang BL, Yao KZ. Effects of intrathecal and i.v. small-dose sufentanil on the median effective dose of intrathecal bupivacaine for caesarean section. Br J Anaesth. 2007;98:792-6.

[78] Braga A de F, Braga FS, Potério GM, et al. Sufentanil added to hyperbaric bupivacaine for subarachnoid block in caesarean section. Eur J Anaesthesiol. 2003;20:631-5.

[79] Demiraran Y, Ozdemir I, Kocaman B, Yucel O. Intrathecal sufentanil (1.5 microg) added to hyperbaric bupivacaine (0.5%) for elective cesarean section provides adequate analgesia without need for pruritus therapy. J Anesth. 2006;20:274-8.

[80] Bang YS, Chung KH, Lee JH, et al. Comparison of clinical effects according to the dosage of sufentanil added to 0.5% hyperbaric bupivacaine for spinal anesthesia in patients undergoing cesarean section. Korean J Anesthesiol. 2012;63:321-6.

[81] Bozdogan Ozyilkan N, Kocum A, Sener M, et al. Comparison of intrathecal levobupivacaine combined with sufentanil, fentanyl, or placebo for elective caesarean section: a prospective, randomized, double-blind, controlled study. Curr Ther Res Clin. Exp. 2013;75:64-70.

[82] Karaman S, Kocabas S, Uyar M, Hayzaran S, Firat V. The effects of sufentanil or morphine added to hyperbaric bupivacaine in spinal anaesthesia for caesarean section. Eur J Anaesthesiol. 2006;23:285-91.

[83] Chen X, Qian X, Fu F, Lu H, Bein B. Intrathecal sufentanil decreases the median effective dose (ED50) of intrathecal hyperbaric ropivacaine for caesarean delivery. Acta Anaesthesiol Scand. 2010;54:284-90.

[84] Qian XW, Chen XZ, Li DB. Low-dose ropivacaine-sufentanil spinal anaesthesia for caesarean delivery: a randomised trial. Int J Obstet Anesth. 2008;17:309-14.

[85] Sun MY, Liao Q, Luo XH, Ouyang W. The optimal dose of intrathecal sufentanil to be added to low-dose intrathecal ropivacaine during anesthesia for cesarean delivery. Saudi Med J. 2011;32:855-7.

[86] Bakhshaei MH, Manuchehrian N, Khoshraftar E, Mohamadipour-Anvary H, Sanatkarfar M. Analgesic effects of intrathecal sufentanil added to lidocaine 5% in elective cesarean section. Acta Med Iran. 2010;48:380-4.

[87] Dahlgren G, Hultstrand C, Jakobsson J, et al. Intrathecal sufentanil, fentanyl, or placebo added to bupivacaine for cesarean section. Anesth Analg. 1997;85:1288-93.

[88] Meininger D, Byhahn C, Kessler P, et al. Intrathecal fentanyl, sufentanil, or placebo combined with hyperbaric mepivacaine 2% for parturients undergoing elective cesarean delivery. Anesth Analg. 2003;96:852-8.

[89] Lee JH, Chung KH, Lee JY, et al. Comparison of fentanyl and sufentanil added to 0.5% hyperbaric bupivacaine for spinal anesthesia in patients undergoing cesarean section. Korean J Anesthesiol. 2011;60:103-8.

[90] Bremerich DH, Fetsch N, Zwissler BC, et al.Comparison of intrathecal bupivacaine and levobupivacaine combined with opioids for caesarean section. Curr Med Res Opin. 2007;23:3047-54.

[91] de Figueiredo Locks G. Incidence of shivering after cesarean section under spinal anesthesia with or without intrathecal sufentanil: a randomized study. Rev Bras Anestesiol. 2012;62:676-84.

[92] Latta KS, Ginsberg B, Barkin RL.Meperidine: a critical review. Am J Ther. 2002;9:53-68.

[93] Ngan Kee WD. Intrathecal pethidine: pharmacology and clinical applications. Anaesth Intensive Care. 1998;26:137-46.

[94] Kafle SK. Intrathecal meperidine for elective caesarean section: a comparison with lidocaine. Can J Anaesth. 1993;40:718-21.

[95] Nguyen Thi TV, Orliaguet G, Ngû TH, Bonnet F. Spinal anesthesia with meperidine as the sole agent for cesarean delivery. Reg Anesth. 1994;19:386-9.

[96] Cheun JK, Kim AR. Intrathecal meperidine as the sole agent for cesarean section. J Korean Med Sci. 1989;4:135-8.

[97] Yu SC, Ngan Kee WD, Kwan AS. Addition of meperidine to bupivacaine for spinal anaesthesia for caesarean section. Br J Anaesth. 2002;88:379-83.

[98] Imarengiaye CO, Asudo FD, Akpoguado DD, et al. Subarachnoid bupivacaine and pethidine for caesarean section: assessment of quality of perioperative analgesia and side effects. Niger Postgrad Med J. 2011;18:200-4.

[99] Farzi F, Mirmansouri A, Forghanparast K, et al. Addition of intrathecal fentanyl or meperidine to lidocaine and epinephrine for spinal anesthesia in elective cesarean delivery. Anesth Pain Med. 2014;4:e14081.

[100] Camann WR, Bader AM. Spinal anesthesia for cesarean delivery with meperidine as the sole agent. Int J Obstet Anesth. 1992;1:156-8.

[101] Vassiliadis RM, Taylor PG. Spinal pethidine for elective caesarean section. Anaesth Intensive Care. 2013;41:113-5.

[102] Jaillon P, Gardin ME, Lecocq B, Richard MO. Pharmacokinetics of nalbuphine in infants, young healthy volunteers, and elderly patients. Clin Pharmacol Ther. 1989;46:226-33.

[103] Errick JK, Heel RC. Nalbuphine. A preliminary review of its pharmacological properties and therapeutic efficacy. Drugs. 1983;26:191-211.

[104] Rawal N, Nuutinen L, Raj PP, et al. Behavioral and histopathologic effects following intrathecal administration of butorphanol, sufentanil, and nalbuphine in sheep. Anesthesiology 1991;75:1025-34.

[105] Schmauss C, Doherty C, Yaksh TL. The analgetic effects of an intrathecally administered partial opiate agonist, nalbuphine hydrochloride. Eur J Pharmacol. 1982;86:1-7.

[106] Fournier R, Van Gessel E, Macksay M, Gamulin Z. Onset and offset of intrathecal morphine versus nalbuphine for postoperative pain relief after total hip replacement. Acta Anaesthesiol Scand. 2000;44:940-5.

[107] Tiwari AK, Tomar GS, Agrawal J. Intrathecal bupivacaine in comparison with a combination of nalbuphine and bupivacaine for subarachnoid block: a randomized prospective double-blind clinical study. Am J Ther. 2013;20:592-5.

[108] Mukherjee A, Pal A, Agrawal J, Mehrotra A, Dawar N. Intrathecal nalbuphine as an adjuvant to subarachnoid block: What is the most effective dose?. Anesth Essays Res. 2011;5:171-5.

[109] Culebras X, Gaggero G, Zatloukal J, Kern C, Marti RA. Advantages of intrathecal nalbuphine, compared with intrathecal morphine, after cesarean delivery: an evaluation of postoperative analgesia and adverse effects. Anesth Analg. 2000;91:601-5.

[110] Yaksh T, Birnbach DJ. Intrathecal nalbuphine after cesarean delivery: are we ready? Anesth Analg. 2000;91:505-8.

[111] Yoon HJ, Jee YS, Hong JY. A comparison of analgesic and side effects of intrathecal morphine, nalbuphine and morphine-nalbuphine mixture for pain relief during a cesarean section. Korean J Anesthesiol. 2002;42:627-33.

[112] Gomaa HM, Mohamed NN, Zoheir HAH, Ali MS. A comparison between post-operative analgesia after intrathecal nalbuphine with bupivacaine and intrathecal fentanyl with bupivacaine after cesarean section. Egypt J Anaesth. 2014;03.008.

[113] Kehl F, Erfkamp S, Roewer N. Respiratory arrest during caesarean section after intrathecal administration of sufentanil in combination with 0.1% bupivacaine 10 ml. Anaesth Intensive Care. 2002;30:698-9.

[114] Katsiris S, Williams S, Leighton BL, Halpern S. Respiratory arrest following intrathecal injection of sufentanil and bupivacaine in a parturient. Can J Anaesth. 1998;45:880-3.

[115] Greenhalgh CA. Respiratory arrest in a parturient following intrathecal injection of sufentanil and bupivacaine. Anaesthesia 1996;51:173-5.

[116] Gehling M, Tryba M. Risks and side-effects of intrathecal morphine combined with spinal anaesthesia: a meta-analysis. Anaesthesia 2009;64:643-51.

[117] Dalchow S, Lubeigt O, Peters G, et al. Transcutaneous carbon dioxide levels and oxygen saturation following caesarean section performed under spinal anaesthesia with intrathecal opioids. Int J Obstet Anesth. 2013;22:217-22.

[118] Tshibangu-N A, Motte-Neuville F, Gepts E, Bailly A, Nguyen T, Hirsoux L. Impact of intrathecal morphine on the tolerance of early feeding after cesarean section. Ann Fr Anesth Reanim. 2010;29:113-6.

[119] Yazigi A, Chalhoub V, Madi-Jebara S, Haddad F, Hayek G. Prophylactic ondansetron is effective in the treatment of nausea and vomiting but not on pruritus after cesarean delivery with intrathecal sufentanil-morphine. J Clin Anesth. 2002;14:183-6.

[120] George RB, Allen TK, Habib AS. Serotonin receptor antagonists for the prevention and treatment of pruritus, nausea, and vomiting in women undergoing cesarean delivery with intrathecal morphine: a systematic review and meta-analysis. Anesth Analg. 2009;109:174-82.

[121] Tamdee D, Charuluxananan S, Punjasawadwong Y, et al. A randomized controlled trial of pentazocine versus ondansetron for the treatment of intrathecal morphine-induced pruritus in patients undergoing cesarean delivery. Anesth Analg. 2009;109:1606-11.

[122] Wu Z, Kong M, Wang N, Finlayson RJ, De Tran QH. Intravenous butorphanol administration reduces intrathecal morphine-induced pruritus after cesarean delivery: a randomized, double-blind, placebo-controlled study. J Anesth. 2012;26:752-7.

[123] Dominguez JE, Habib AS. Prophylaxis and treatment of the side-effects of neuraxial morphine analgesia following cesarean delivery. Curr Opin Anaesthesiol. 2013;26:288-95.

[124] Sayyid SS, Jabbour DG, Baraka AS. Hypothermia and excessive sweating following intrathecal morphine in a parturient undergoing cesarean delivery. Reg Anesth Pain Med. 2003;28:140-3.

[125] Hess PE, Snowman CE, Wang J. Hypothermia after cesarean delivery and its reversal with lorazepam. Int J Obstet Anesth. 2005;14:279-83.

[126] Fischer MO, Dequiré PM, Kalem A, Gérard JL, Plaud B. Hypothermia after spinal anaesthesia: implication of morphine? Ann Fr Anesth Reanim. 2006;25:296-8.

[127] Valente A, Ciano F, Suppa E, Draisci G. Hypothermia after cesarean section with combined spinal-epidural anesthesia and postoperative epidural analgesia. Int J Obstet Anesth. 2008;17:78.

[128] Ryan KF, Price JW, Warriner CB, Choi PT. Persistent hypothermia after intrathecal morphine: case report and literature review. Can J Anaesth. 2012;59:384-8.

[129] Harkouk H, de Préville G, Benhamou D. Hypothermia after intrathecal morphine for caesarean delivery: Another case report. Ann Fr Anesth Reanim. 2013;32:53-5.

[130] Christiansson L. Update on adjuvants in regional anaesthesia. Periodicum Bilogorum 2009;111:161-70.

[131] Whizar LV. Intrathecal clonidine as adjuvant for labor analgesia, spinal anesthesia, and postoperative analgesia in caesarean section. J Anesth Crit Care Open Access 2014;1:0005.

[132] Bhure A, Kalita N, Ingley P, Gadkari CP. Comparison of different doses of clonidine as an adjuvant to intrathecal bupivacaine for spinal anesthesia and postoperative an-

algesia in patients undergoing caesarian section. People's J Scient Research 2012;5:19-23.

[133] Eisenach JC, Castro MI, Dewan DM, Rose JC. Epidural clonidine analgesia in obstetrics: sheep studies. Anesthesiology 1989;70:51-56.

[134] Eisenach JC, Dewan DM. Intrathecal clonidine in obstetrics: sheep studies. Anesthesiology 1990;72:663-668.

[135] Filos KS, Goudas LC, Patroni O, Polyzou V. Intrathecal clonidine as a sole analgesic for pain relief after cesarean section. Anesthesiology 1992;77: 267-74.

[136] Filos KS, Goudas LC, Patroni O, Polyzou V. Hemodynamic and analgesic profile after intrathecal clonidine in humans. A dose-response study. Anesthesiology 1994;81:591-601.

[137] Paech MJ, Pavy TJ, Orlikowski CE, et al. Postcesarean analgesia with spinal morphine, clonidine, or their combination. Anesth Analg. 2004;98:1460-1466.

[138] Khezri MB, Rezaei M, Delkhosh Reihany M, Haji Seid Javadi E. Comparison of postoperative analgesic effect of intrathecal clonidine and fentanyl added to bupivacaine in patients undergoing cesarean section: a prospective randomized double-blind study. Pain Res Treat. 2014;2014:513628.

[139] Singh R, Gupta D, Jain A. The effect of addition of intrathecal clonidine to hyperbaric bupivacaine on postoperative pain after lower segment caesarean section: A randomized control trial. Saudi J Anaesth. 2013;7:283-290.

[140] van Tuijl I, van Klei WA, van der Werff DB, Kalkman CJ. The effect of addition of intrathecal clonidine to hyperbaric bupivacaine on postoperative pain and morphine requirements after caesarean section: a randomized controlled trial. Br J Anaesth. 2006;97:365-70.

[141] Sachan P, Kumar N, Sharma J P. Intrathecal clonidine with hyperbaric bupivacaine administered as a mixture and sequentially in caesarean section: A randomised controlled study. Indian J Anaesth 2014;58:287-92.

[142] Reves JG, Fragen RJ, Vinik HR, Greenblatt DJ. Midazolam: pharmacology and uses. Anesthesiology. 1985;62:310-24.

[143] Johansen MJ, Gradert TL, Satterfield WC, et al. Safety of continuous intrathecal midazolam infusion in the sheep model. Anesth Analg. 2004;98:1528-35.

[144] Prakash S, Joshi N, Gogia AR, Prakash S, Singh R.Analgesic efficacy of two doses of intrathecal midazolam with bupivacaine in patients undergoing cesarean delivery. Reg Anesth Pain Med. 2006;31:221-6.

[145] Karbasfrushan A, Farhadi K, Amini-Saman J, Bazargan-Hejazi S, Ahmadi A. Effect of intrathecal midazolam in the severity of pain in cesarean section: a randomized controlled trail. Iran Red Crescent Med J. 2012;14:276-82.

[146] Salimi A, Nejad RA, Safari F, et al. Reduction in labor pain by intrathecal midazolam as an adjunct to sufentanil. Korean J Anesthesiol. 2014;66:204-9.

[147] Albrecht E, Kern C, Kirkham KR. The safety profile of neuraxial magnesium has not been properly addressed. Br J Anaesth. 2014;112:173-4.

[148] Mebazaa MS, Ouerghi S, Frikha N, et al. Is magnesium sulfate by the intrathecal route efficient and safe? Ann Fr Anesth Reanim. 2011;30:47-50.

[149] Ozdogan L, Sastim H, Ornek D, et al. Neurotoxic effects of intrathecal magnesium sulphate. Braz J Anesthesiol. 2013;63:139-43.

[150] Arcioni R, Palmisani S, Tigano S, et al. Combined intrathecal and epidural magnesium sulfate supplementation of spinal anesthesia to reduce post-operative analgesic requirements: a prospective, randomized, double-blind, controlled trial in patients undergoing major orthopedic surgery. Acta Anaesthesiol Scand. 2007;51:482-9.

[151] Khalili G, Janghorbani M, Sajedi P, Ahmadi G. Effects of adjunct intrathecal magnesium sulfate to bupivacaine for spinal anesthesia: a randomized, double-blind trial in patients undergoing lower extremity surgery. J Anesth. 2011;25:892-7.

[152] Ozalevli M, Cetin TO, Unlugenc H, Guler T, Isik G. The effect of adding intrathecal magnesium sulphate to bupivacaine-fentanyl spinal anaesthesia. Acta Anaesthesiol Scand. 2005;49:1514-9.

[153] Yousef AA, Amr YM. The effect of adding magnesium sulphate to epidural bupivacaine and fentanyl in elective caesarean section using combined spinal-epidural anaesthesia: a prospective double blind randomised study. Int J Obstet Anesth. 2010;19:401-4.

[154] Sun J, Wu X, Xu X, et al. A comparison of epidural magnesium and/or morphine with bupivacaine for postoperative analgesia after cesarean section. Int J Obstet Anesth. 2012;21:310-6.

[155] Ghrab BE, Maatoug M, Kallel N, et al. Does combination of intrathecal magnesium sulfate and morphine improve postcaesarean section analgesia? Ann Fr Anesth Reanim. 2009;28:454-9.

[156] Jabalameli M, Pakzadmoghadam SH. Adding different doses of intrathecal magnesium sulfate for spinal anesthesia in the cesarean section: A prospective double blind randomized trial. Adv Biomed Res. 2012;1:7

[157] Malleeswaran S, Panda N, Mathew P, Bagga R. A randomised study of magnesium sulphate as an adjuvant to intrathecal bupivacaine in patients with mild preeclampsia undergoing caesarean section. Int J Obstet Anesth. 2010;19:161-6.

[158] Faiz SH, Rahimzadeh P, Imani F, Bakhtiari A. Intrathecal injection of magnesium sulfate: shivering prevention during cesarean section: a randomized, double-blinded, controlled study. Korean J Anesthesiol. 2013;65:293-8.

[159] Unlugenc H, Ozalevli M, Gunduz M, et al. Comparison of intrathecal magnesium, fentanyl, or placebo combined with bupivacaine 0.5% for parturients undergoing elective cesarean delivery. Acta Anaesthesiol Scand. 2009;53:346-53.

Chapter 5

Intrathecal Clonidine as Spinal Anaesthesia Adjuvant — Is there a Magical Dose?

Víctor M. Whizar-Lugo, Juan C. Flores-Carrillo and Susana Preciado-Ramírez

Additional information is available at the end of the chapter

http://dx.doi.org/10.5772/58712

1. Introduction

Clonidine was synthesized in 1962 as nasal decongestant, and marketed as antihypertensive in 1972. Bloor and Flacke in 1982 [1] demonstrated in mongrel dogs that intravenous clonidine 5 and 20 μg/kg decreased halothane MAC by 42% and 48% respectively. Since then, clonidine has been used by anaesthesiologists as an anaesthetic adjunct to provide increased perioperative cardiovascular and sympathoadrenal stability, to enhance general and regional anaesthesia, as well as sedation and analgesia. [2, 3] In 1999, dexmedetomidine, a novel selective and specific alpha2 agonist, was approved for postoperative sedation in intensive care patients, and has also been investigated in general anaesthesia, regional anaesthesia and pain treatment. Basic research in animals and clinical studies in humans performed with epidural clonidine have shown its analgesic effects, with less side effects than any other neuroaxial anaesthesia adjuvant. Similar results were also obtained with intrathecal injection of clonidine. Due to the short duration of analgesic action by the latter route, the extradural administration is the most studied. Epidural administration of clonidine has been widely utilized; indeed, the FDA has only approved peridural use of clonidine infusion in chronic pain patients. There are many publications with epidural clonidine for intraoperative surgical pain as an adjunct to general anaesthesia and epidural anaesthesia, postoperative pain, pediatrics, and labour analgesia. It has been used alone, or in combination with local anaesthetics, opioids, in bolus, or by continuous infusion.

Intrathecal administration of clonidine is an interesting alternative route of administration. As an alpha2 agonist, spinal injected clonidine prolongs sensory and motor block, increases sedation and may potentiate hypotension and bradycardia. It has been used in high (> 150 μg), low (< 150 μg) and small (< 75 μg) doses. High doses 150, 300 and 450 μg produce dose dependent analgesia, enhance spinal anaesthesia, with relative hemodynamic stability. Furthermore, doses of 15 and 30 μg in addition to spinal local anaesthetics provide better sensory and motor block compared to local anaesthetics alone. [4, 5]

The optimal dose of spinal clonidine remains unknown. For short ambulatory procedures 15 to 75 μg added to local anaesthetics enhance spinal anaesthesia without negative impact on home discharge criteria. For short-stay or longer hospitalization surgeries, doses from 150 up to 450 μg of clonidine as adjuvant for any local anaesthetics are safe, prolongs motor and sensory block, and reduces the need of postoperative opioids.

This chapter updates current data on dose-response relationship of subarachnoid clonidine when added as adjunct to spinal local anaesthetics and/or spinal opioids in different clinical surgery scenarios, as well as for postoperative analgesia and labour pain.

2. Spinal additives

Spinal adjuvant drugs have been used since the beginning of subarachnoid anaesthesia. Adrenaline, an alpha2 agonist, was the first drug used to enhance duration of spinal anaesthesia, and morphine was the first opioid injected with eucaine in the lumbar spinal space to relieve vertebral pain. [6] After the first article on spinal analgesia using opioids written by Yaksh and Rudy in 1976, [7] the neuroaxial route to inject opioids as adjuvants drugs grew logarithmically. Morphine, fentanyl, sufentanyl and many more agonist opioids have proven their safety and efficacy to decrease the dose of local anaesthetics, to facilitate a faster recovery, and effective postoperative analgesia. There are many receptors which modulates spinal pain response; however, there are only few FDA approved drugs to be used via subarachnoid as adjuvants or sole medications.

Many drugs have being injected into the spinal or peridural space in order to provide analgesia and/or to enhance neuraxial anaesthesia. Nowadays, opioids are the more frequently used spinal additives, but their side effects may limit its use; pruritus, urinary retention and late respiratory depression. There are studies with intrathecal adjuvants that have not been approved to be used in spinal anaesthesia: midazolam, ketamine, neostigmine, magnesium sulphate, calcium channel blockers, nonsteroidal anti-inflammatory, dexmedetomidine, tizanidine, etcetera.

3. Alpha2 adrenergic agonist drugs

Alpha2 agonist medications are used as adjuvants in anaesthesia and analgesia. They can be prescribed orally, transdermally, intravenously, perineuraly, or through the neuroaxial route. Beside analgesia and sedation, they decrease sympathetic tone and attenuate the stress response to anaesthesia and surgery. Although adrenaline was the first alpha2 agonist used intrathecally, it is no longer recommended. Nowadays, clonidine is the most used alpha2

http://dx.doi.org/10.5772/58712

agonist in neuroaxial anaesthesia, even though dexmedetomidine has also recently been studied for epidural and spinal anaesthesia adjuvant. Clonidine acts as a selective partial agonist with a ratio of 200:1, whereas dexmedetomidine is highly selective with a ratio of 1600:1. Tizanidine, 5-bromo-N-[4, 5-dihydro-1H-imidazol-2-yl)-6-quinoxalinamine (UK-14, 304], and moxonidine are other alpha2 agonists with a potential neuroaxial use. [8, 9, 10, 11] More than 90 patents have been deposited recently regarding different methods of alpha2 modulation (use of agonists or antagonists, nucleic acids and polypeptides) for diagnosis, prognosis and treatment of disorders involving this receptors.

4. Clonidine

This prototypical alpha2 adrenergic receptor agonist was developed in the early 1960s. It is an imidazoline derivative that exists as a mesomeric compound. It has a molecular weight of 266.56, chemical name is Benzenamine, 2, 6-dichloro-N-2-imidazolindinylidene monohydrochloride and 2-[[2, 6-dichlorophenyl) imino] imidazolidine monohidrochloride. Figure 1 shows its structural formula (C9H9Cl2N3 HCl). Clonidine stimulates alpha2 adrenoreceptors in the brain and spinal cord, resulting in reduction of sympathetic outflow from the central nervous system and in decreased in peripheral resistance, renal vascular resistance, plasma renin activity, heart rate, cardiac output, and blood pressure. Normal postural reflexes are intact; therefore, orthostatic symptoms are mild and infrequent. Plasmatic level of clonidine peaks in approximately 3 to 5 hours and the plasma half-life ranges from 12 to 16 hours. The half-life increases up to 41 hours in patients with severe renal impairment. Following oral administration, approximately 75% is bioavailable in men, about 40-60% of the absorbed dose recovered unchanged in the urine in 24 hours. About 50% of the absorbed dose is metabolized in the liver. Severe adverse side effects are infrequent, and well tolerated in most patients. Sedation and dry mouth are the most common side effects, and are usually related to dose and length of administration. [12, 13]

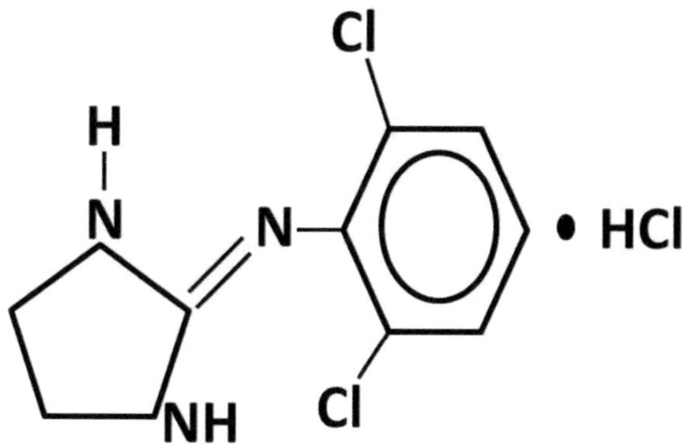

Figure 1. Structural formula of clonidine

5. Mechanisms of action of spinal clonidine

It has been shown that epidural and spinal administration of clonidine in surgical patients enhances quality and duration of neuroaxial anaesthesia, reduces dose of local anaesthetics as well as others neuroaxial additives such opioids. It also produces a short period of postoperative analgesia, and lowers the dose of systemic postoperative analgesics.

G-protein-coupled receptors (GPCRs) are the largest and most diverse superfamily of membrane receptors responsible for signaling between cells and tissues, mediating most cellular responses to hormones and neurotransmitters, playing important physiological roles in homeostasis. They are a major drug targets. The alpha2 adrenoceptors are membrane proteins belonging to these superfamily GPCRs, that form a group of 3 to 4 gene polymorphic products, that mediate major central nervous system actions of norepinephrine and epinephrine, including control of mood state, arousal, endocrine function, autonomic and somatic motor outflows, and modulation sensory inputs, including pain. The alpha2 adrenoceptors are located presynaptically and regulates the release of the neurotransmitter; they are also present in postsynaptical locations.

Three distinct subtypes have been described, characterized and cloned; alpha2A, alpha2B, and alpha2C. [14, 15, 16, 17] There is a fourth receptor called alfa2D that has been described and their functions are still not known, although it appears that this receptor alfa2D is in fact, an alpha2A-D subtype; the alpha2A in humans and the alpha2D in rats. [18]

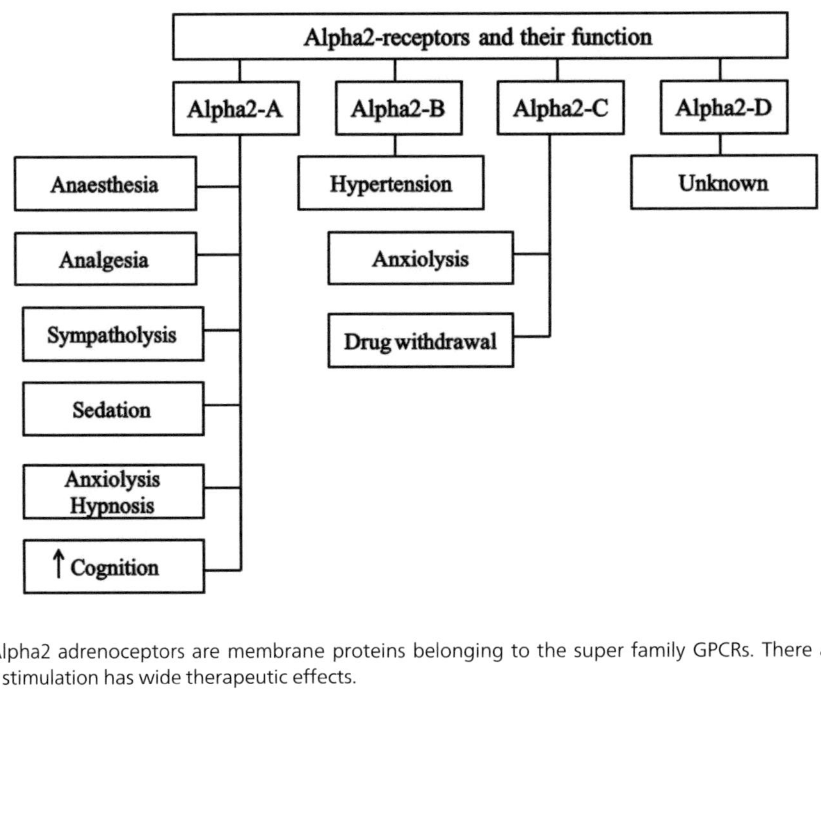

Figure 2. Alpha2 adrenoceptors are membrane proteins belonging to the super family GPCRs. There are four subtypes. Their stimulation has wide therapeutic effects.

http://dx.doi.org/10.5772/58712

The anatomic site of action of the alpha2 agonists involves specific receptors of the spinal dorsal horn and supraspinaly in the nucleus coereleus in the pons. [19, 20, 21, 22] While the mechanism and location of action of the sedative effect of these compounds are due to the hyperpolarization of excitable neurons localized in the nucleous coereleus, the analgesic effect of these drugs is not completely understood, and have a complex mechanism. Alpha 2 agonists induce analgesia by acting in different places; brain, brain stem, spinal cord and peripheral nerves. Their supraspinaly analgesic mechanism in the locus coereleus is probably by transduction, while in the spinal cord is likely related to activation of the descending medullospinal noradrenergic pathways or to the reduction of spinal sympathetic outflow at presynaptic ganglionic sites. Clonidine suppresses the generation of action potentials in tonic-firing spinal dorsal horn neurons. This may be explained, in part, by an interaction with voltage-gated Na^+ and K^+ currents.

Clonidine also acts synergistically with local anaesthetics because of its action of opening potassium channels.

6. Spinal interactions between alfa2 agonists and opioids

It is an uncommon clinical practice to combine alpha2 agonists and opioids in spinal anaesthesia to either enhance local anaesthetic effects or to provide postoperative analgesia. This technique is based on the spinal synergism between these two drugs. When morphine and clonidine are co-administered intrathecally, the resulting antinociception is greater than expected if the drug responses were additive; thus, a synergistic interaction is present. [23, 24] For the most part, the underlying molecular synergy mechanisms are not known, although some studies have identified both the delta and the mu-opioid receptors as candidate receptors capable of interacting synergistically with alpha 2A agonists. Roerig et al [25] found in rats that interactions between opioid and adrenergic agonists in mouse spinal cord were mediated by delta and alpha2 receptor subtypes, the synergistic interaction between morphine and alpha2 adrenergic agonists may involve action at delta opioid receptors, and antagonist action on these drug interactions is intrincated. Stone and coworkers, [26] in a genetically modified mouse line expressing a point mutation (D79N) in the alpha2A adrenergic receptor investigated the role of the alpha2A receptor in alpha2 agonist-evoked analgesia and adrenergic-opioid synergy. They were able to demonstrate that the alpha2A subtype receptor is the primary mediator of alpha2 adrenergic spinal analgesia and is necessary for analgesic synergy with opioids, and concluded that combination therapies targeting the alpha2A receptor and opioid receptors may be useful in maximizing the analgesic efficacy of opioids while decreasing total dose requirements. Although others have found that the alpha2C adrenergic receptor subtype contributes to this synergy, [27] Chabot-Doré and coworkers [28] confirmed that although other opioid receptors can interact synergistically with alpha2 receptors agonists, Delta opioid receptor is sufficient for spinal opioid-adrenergic interactions. Protein kinase is needed for this analgesic synergy. [29]

Analgesic synergy between opioid and alpha2 adrenergic agonists is potentially beneficial by increasing efficacy and/or reducing the total drug required to produce sufficient pain relief, and undesired side effects can be minimized.

7. Safety of spinal clonidine

Neurotoxicity has not been reported following the use of intrathecal clonidine and generally the drug is considered to be safe in this regard. Although subarachnoid administration of clonidine has not been approved by the FDA or any other regulatory agency in the world, there are experimental studies that have demonstrated its safety and efficacy when used by this route. Continuous administration of spinal clonidine in Wistar rats during 14 days failed to demonstrate neurotoxic damage. [30] Erddivanli and coworkers injected male Sprague-Dawley rats [31] with 3 μg and 10 μg of intrathecal dexmedetomidine added to bupivacaine; they found no apparent pathohistological changes 24 hours after a single injection. In male Kunming mice 1 to 3 μg of dexmedetomidine displayed a robust analgesia via a alpha2-receptor in a dose dependent manner and no significant pathological impacts on the spinal cord were noticed, with a potential protective effects of lidocaine induced neural cell damage. [32] In postnatal rats spinal clonidine produces age and dose-dependent analgesia, without signs of spinal cord toxicity, even at doses bigger than required for analgesia. [33]

8. Clinical use of spinal clonidine

To enhance spinal anaesthesia and postoperative pain control clonidine can be injected in the subarachnoid space as an adjuvant drug to opioids or local anaesthetics. A systematic review by Elia et al [34] including 1, 445 patients using a wide variety of spinal clonidine doses as adjuvant to subarachnoid bupivacaine, mepivacaine, prilocaine, or tetracaine found that 15 to 150 μg prolonged in a linear, dose-dependent manner, the time to 2 segment regression (range of means, 14 to 75 minutes) and also delayed the regression time to L2 dermatome (range of means, 11 to 128 minutes). The time to first analgesic request (median 101 minutes, range 35 to 310] and motor block (median 47 minutes, range 6 to 131] was extended with no relation to dose. There were fewer episodes of intraoperative pain with clonidine (relative risk, 0.24; 95% confidence interval [CI], 0.09-0.64; number needed to treat, 13] but more episodes of arterial hypotension (relative risk, 1.81; 95% CI 1.44-2.28; number needed to harm, 8] without evidence of dose-responsiveness. The risk of bradycardia was unchanged.

Side effects of intrathecal clonidine include sedation, hypotension and a reduction of the heart rate. Especially in post-surgical patients these circumstance warrants specific attention.

The following paragraphs discuss spinal clonidine use in different anaesthetic and surgical scenarios, as well as in the management of postoperative and labour pain.

http://dx.doi.org/10.5772/58712

9. Ambulatory settings

Spinal anaesthesia side effects are a major concern in some patients and physicians and may be reluctant to use this technique in ambulatory surgery. [35] Nowadays there are many articles showing that spinal anaesthesia is a safe and effective technique in this clinical scenario. There is an special interest to use adjuncts drugs such clonidine in order to decrease local anaesthetic dose to promptly achieve a recovery profile. [36]

Several investigations in patients undergoing knee arthroscopy have shown that low doses of clonidine [15 up to 45 μg) added to low doses of intrathecal hyperbaric bupivacaine [5-6 mg) improves the quality of anaesthesia, prolong the motor block, without affecting time to home discharge in outpatients. [37] In 60 ambulatory patients undergoing knee arthroscopy Marrivirta et al [38] added 75 μg clonidine to 6 mg spinal hyperbaric bupivacaine vs. 6 mg bupivacaine alone. These researchers found that motor block was prolonged in those patients who received clonidine without affecting home-readiness. Also these patients needed more vasopressors and had less postoperative pain. Adding clonidine 15 μg to 8 mg of isobaric spinal ropivacaine [39] did not prolonged motor or sensory blockade, but enhanced anaesthesia quality for knee arthroscopy. Bigger doses such 75 μg produced significantly longer sensory and motor blockade [195 ± 40 min and 164 ± 38 min; $p < 0.05$], but associated with sedation and hypotension.

In our practice we have good results with doses of 45-150 μg. These doses of spinal clonidine favor the reduction of local anaesthetics doses and do not prolong the recovery time of our outpatients.

10. General surgery and urologic procedures

Numerous surgical procedures of the abdominal wall, abdominopelvic cavity, and retroperitoneum can be performed under single injection of local anaesthetics in the spinal space. For prolonged cases the use of adjuvant drugs improves the quality and increases the duration of the subarachnoid block. Clonidine has been used successfully in various surgical procedures of the abdomen and pelvis. Intrathecal clonidine 15, 30, 45 and 75 μg alone, or added to opioids expand spinal anaesthesia sensory block and duration of motor block, and also provided prolonged postoperative analgesia. In a randomized study [40] of 73 patients ASA physical status I and II undergoing gynecological abdominal surgery with spinal bupivacaine 15 mg, the authors compared clonidine 30 μg, sufentanyl 10 μg, clonidine 15μg plus sufentanil 15 μg versus a control group. Sensory block to pinprick at 10 min was higher for clonidine and sufentanil/clonidine groups compared to the control group ($p < 0.02$]. Anaesthetic time (Bromage score 2] was also longer for clonidine and sufentanil/clonidine groups compared to the control and sufentanil groups ($p < 0.05$]. Time to first rescue analgesics was shorter in the control group compared to the other groups ($p < 0.02$]. The dose of intramuscular diclofenac in 24 hours was higher in the control group compared to all other groups ($p < 0.05$]. The incidence of adverse effects and ephedrine consumption were similar among groups. Clonidine 75 μg associated with 17.5 mg hyperbaric bupivacaine 0.5% for lower abdominal surgeries [41] with high level spinal anaesthesia (T4] induced a higher incidence of arterial hypotension but prolongs sensory block and postoperative analgesia similar to clonidine 45 μg. In lower abdomen surgeries, Yoganarasimha and coworkers [42] compared intrathecal clonidine 75 μg versus intrathecal neostigmine 50 μg as adjuvant drugs for spinal anaesthesia 0.5% hyperbaric bupivacaine 12.5 mg; analgesia was prolonged significantly with clonidine [362 ± 36 min) compared with neostigmine [300 ± 25 min)(p < 0.05]. No serious adverse effects were noted perioperatively in either group. In an interesting clinical study with 60 patients undergoing right colon resection under general anaesthesia, preoperative intrathecal clonidine was superior to bupivacaine to prevent postoperative secondary hyperalgesia; [43] the authors compared the effect of clonidine 300 μg versus bupivacaine 10 mg intrathecally versus saline (control group): morphine needs patient controlled postoperative analgesia were less in the clonidine group [31.5±12 versus 91±25.5 and 43±15 mg, respectively, in groups clonidine, saline, and bupivacaine: p < 0.05 at 72 postoperative hours). The area of mechanical hyperalgesia at 72 h was 3±5 cm^2 in the clonidine group versus 90±30 and 35±20 cm^2 in the saline and bupivacaine groups (p < 0.05]. After 6 months, fewer patients in the clonidine group experienced residual pain than in the saline group [0 of 20 versus 6 of 20, p < 0.05]. In laparoscopic procedures done under bupivacaine spinal anaesthesia, clonidine 30 μg produced good sedation, intra and postoperative analgesia, and abolished shoulder tip pain during the procedures. [44] For inguinal hernioplasthy [45, 46] adding clonidine 15 or 30 μg to small doses of hyperbaric bupivacaine enhance spinal anaesthesia, prolongs the time to first analgesic request, and decreases postoperative pain, compared with bupivacaine alone. Thirty μg clonidine was associated with higher incidence and duration of hypotension than 15 μg of clonidine.

Some research has shown the usefulness of intrathecal clonidine in urology procedures, although there are some controversies. In a controlled, prospective, double-blind investigation with patients undergoing elective transurethral resection of bladder tumours under spinal anaesthesia [47] the authors found that adding clonidine 75 μg to prilocaine 75 mg increased the duration of sensory and motor block and reduced the need for additional postoperative analgesics by providing excellent analgesia for about 8 hours during recovery period. In a similar study, 25 μg spinal clonidine improved bupivacaine spinal anaesthesia: shorter time to achieve complete motor block and sensory block at T9 level, with longer postoperative analgesia. [48] In 60 patients undergoing transurethral resection of prostate or bladder tumors Kanazi et al [49] compared clonidine 30 μg, versus dexmedetomidine 3 μg added to 12 mg spinal hyperbaric bupivacaine, versus bupivacaine alone. Patients treated with alpha2 agonists had a significantly shorter onset time of motor block and significantly longer sensory and motor regression times than patients who only received local anaesthetic. The mean time of sensory regression to the S1 segment was 303 ±75 min for those injected with dexmedetomidine, 272 ±38 min in the group who received clonidine and 190±48 min in patients with bupivacaine alone (bupivacaine versus dexmedetomidine and bupivacaine versus clonidine, p< 0.001]. The regression of motor block to Bromage 0 was 250 ±76 min, 216±35 min, and 163±47 min respectively (bupivacaine versus dexmedetomidine and bupivacaine versus clonidine, p< 0.001]. The onset and regression times were not significantly different between patients treated with the alpha2 agonists. The mean arterial pressure, heart rate and level of sedation were similar in the three groups intra-operatively and post-operatively. Andrieu and his group [50] compared intrathecal morphine 4μg/kg without or with clonidine 4μg/kg, or PCA in patients undergoing radical retropubic prostatectomy under general anaesthesia with sevorane-N2O. Adding clonidine to spinal morphine reduced intraoperative use of sufentanil, prolonged time until first request for PCA rescue, and added prolonged analgesia at rest and during coughing.

In contrast with previous mentioned studies, Larsen et al [51] compared 75 μg versus 150 μg of clonidine added to 80 mg mepivacaine 4%, versus spinal mepivacaine alone in patients who had transurethral surgery and found that clonidine had no effect on the onset time, spread or intensity of subarachnoid anaesthesia. The higher dose prolonged the duration of sensory block by 50 minutes and the duration of motor block by 40 minutes, while 75 μg had no significant effect. Heart rate and mean arterial pressure were significantly reduced in both clonidine groups when compared to plain mepivacaine. There was no significant reduction in postoperative analgesic demand. They do not recommend the routine addition of clonidine for spinal anaesthesia with local anaesthetics. There is a reported case of late respiratory depression (16 h after spinal block) in a 70 year old man undergoing prostatic adenomectomy done under spinal anaesthesia with 10 mg bupivacaine, 30 μg clonidine and 100 μg morphine. Intrathecal mixture of morphine-clonidine in older patients must be careful monitored. [52]

10.1. Orthopaedic

Postoperative pain following orthopaedic surgeries has been shown to be a significant negative factor that delay patient recovery and contributes to serious complications. It may also result in larger use of healthcare resources and ultimately lead to poor outcomes. The utilization of multimodal pain management following large orthopaedic surgeries like total joint arthroplasty, total knee replacement, or spinal surgery has positively affected the quality of postoperative care, reduced surgical pain, and decreased the magnitude of opioid consumption and subsequent dose-related complications. Multimodal spinal anaesthesia-analgesia including spinal clonidine is safe and may reduce hospital stay, decrease postoperative complications, and increase patient satisfaction.

In a dose-response prospective study, Strebel et al [53] compared three doses of clonidine (37.5, 75 and 150 μg) added to spinal 0.5% bupivacaine 18 mg in 80 orthopaedics patients. Duration of sensory block (regression below level L1) was increased in patients receiving intrathecal clonidine: 311±101 min in 37.5 μg (+8%), 325 ±69 min in 75 μg (+13%), and 337±78 min in those patients who received 150 μg (+17%) (estimated parameter for dose 0.23 [95% confidence interval-0.05-0.50]). versus control group 288 ±62 min. Time to first analgesic request was also prolonged: 343 ±75 min (+16%), 381±117 min (+29%), and 445±136 min (+51%) (estimated parameter for dose 1.02 [95% confidence interval 0.59-1.45]), respectively compared to control group 295±80 min. Hemodynamic stability was maintained and they found no differences in sedation level. van Tuijl and coworkers [37] investigated the effect of 0, 15 and 30 μg of clonidine added to 5 mg hyperbaric bupivacaine on the duration of motor block, analgesia and ability to void after knee arthroscopy. They found that clonidine increased motor block duration by 25 and 34 min respectively. They also found better analgesic quality, and the mean time for spontaneous voiding was increased up to 18 and 44 min respectively. Amaranto and Berrío demonstrated that spinal clonidine 2 μg/kg added to hyperbaric lidocaine in orthopaedic cases enhance anaesthesia quality, significantly prolonged post operative analgesia, with early motor recovery and minimal side effects. [54] In adolescents scheduled for lower extremities orthopaedic surgery under spinal anaesthesia with isobaric 0.5% bupivacaine added with clonidine 1 μg/kg prolonged duration of sensory and motor block, produced extended spinal postoperative analgesia by 120 min, without severe side effects. [55] Spinal sufentanil 75 μg alone, or added with epinephrine 200 μg, or clonidine 30 μg after total hip replacement results in good analgesia with similar onset and duration of action, and minor side effects. [56] Compared with intrathecal dexmedetomidine, clonidine had a similar results in patients undergoing lower limb surgery with spinal bupivacaine; Mahendru et al [57] conducted a prospective study adding clonidine 30 μg, vs. dexmedetomidine 5 μg, vs. fentanyl 25 μg to 12.5 mg spinal hyperbaric bupivacaine in cases of lower limb surgeries. They discovered that dexmedetomidine prolonged significantly sensory and motor block compared to clonidine, fentanyl and bupivacaine alone. The mean time of two segment sensory block regression was 147±21 min with dexmedetomidine, 117±22 with clonidine, 119±23 in those patients receiving fentanyl, and 102±17 in bupivacaine alone ($p > 0.0001$). The regression time of motor block to reach modified Bromage 0 was 275±25, 199±26, 196±27, 161±20 respectively ($p > 0.0001$). Hemodynamic stability was conserved. In patients 60 years or older undergoing lower extremity orthopaedic surgeries, intrathecally clonidine 15 μg or 30 μg with 9 mg hyperbaric bupivacaine, significantly potentiated the sensory block levels and duration of analgesia without affecting the trend of systolic blood pressure as compared to bupivacaine alone. Clonidine in doses of 30 μg however facilitated the ascent of sensory level block to unexpectedly higher dermatomes for a longer time. [58] Spinal postoperative analgesia can be improved by epidural infusion of 40 μg/h^{-1} mixed with ropivacaine 4 mg/h^{-1} in patients undergoing hip arthroplasty. [59]

Some studies have found conflicting data which showed that spinal clonidine is not a useful adjuvant for postoperative analgesia in orthopedic major surgery. Gehling et al [60] evaluated 45 patients undergoing hip or knee replacement under 15 mg bupivacaine spinal anaesthesia and found a mean time until first opioid request was for placebo 10.3±7.9 h, for 0.1 mg morphine 23.0±3.9 h and for 0.1 mg morphine+50 μg clonidine 21±6.9 h, respectively. Co-administration of pethidine 0.75 mg/kg^{-1} and clonidine 75 μg provided good intraoperative anaesthesia for total hip replacement, but similar to plain isobaric 0.5% bupivacaine. [61]

11. Obstetrics

The role of the anesthesiologist in obstetrics has many responsibilities; labour analgesia, anesthesia for vaginal delivery, anaesthesia for cesarean section, anaesthesia for non-obstetric surgeries during pregnancy, and postoperative analgesia. A comprehensive labour analgesia program has to include newer procedures and ajuvant drugs to facilitate ambulation, excellent pain relief, patient comfort and safety for the mother-fetus binomial. [62, 63, 64] Spinal clonidine has been used for labour analgesia, to enhance spinal anaesthesia during cesarean section, and for postoperative pain relief. Its use tends to be more frequent in this field, since it reduces opioids doses, and thus the side effects such as emesis and maternal pruritus, and the possibility of respiratory depression secondary to rostral opioid distribution. Theoretically, it could also reduce the fetal bradycardia.

Labour analgesia. There are many advances in the pharmacology of labour analgesia focused on alternatives mechanisms to target spinal pain receptors, and the efficacy and safety of old and new drugs and techniques; i.v. remifentanyl for patient controlled analgesia, low dose of diluted local anaesthetics, addition of neuraxial adjuvants like opioids, neostigmine, and clonidine. [65, 66, 67, 68]

Most studied doses of intrathecal clonidine for labour analgesia range from 15 to 45 μg mixed with opioids and/or local anaesthetics. In a preliminary open-label protocol done in France by Mercier and coworkers [69] comparing sufentanil 5 μg+clonidine 30 μg versus sufentanil 5 μg alone injected intrathecally to alleviate pain during the first stage of labour, the authors demonstrated that clonidine potentiate labour analgesia and side effects such hypotension, maternal pruritus and sedation were similar in both groups. In a second research, the same group [70] studied 53 nulliparous women in painful labour using the same doses, but followed by 5 mg of epidural bupivacaine. In this study the duration of analgesia was longer in the sufentanil-clonidine group versus sufentanil alone [125±46 versus 97±30 min, p=0.007]. There were more incidents of hypotension and ephedrine needs in those patients who received sufentanil and clonidine. The incidence of fetal heart rate abnormalities during the first 30 min after spinal injection was similar in both groups [17% versus 19%). No parturient had motor blockade. Gautier et al [71] found that 30 μg of intrathecal clonidine plus 2.5 or 5 μg intrathecal sufentanil increased the duration of labour analgesia during the first stage without undesirable maternal or fetal effects. Labbene et al. [72] added clonidine 15 μg to 2.5 mg isobaric bupivacaine and 5 μg sufentanil during combined spinal-epidural analgesia resulting in extended duration of analgesia without increasing side effects. In nonobstetrical patient doses of 25 to 30 μg of clonidine augmented duration of postoperative analgesia, so smaller dose of clonidine may be effective in the obstetric population.

Chiari et al from Austria [73] did the first study using spinal clonidine as a sole drug for labour analgesia; in 36 parturients with < 6 cm cervical dilation; they compared 50, 100, and 200 μg intrathecal clonidine and found that labour pain was significantly reduced in all patients, analgesia duration was significantly longer with 200 μg (median 143; range 75-210 min), with 100 μg (median 118; range 60-180 min) and using 50 μg (median 45; range 25-150 min). Hypotension was associated with 200 μg and the need of intravenous ephedrine more often than in the other groups.

There are controversies in the use of spinal clonidine for labour analgesia as some researchers have found a higher frequency of maternal hypotension, foetal arrhythmia, and worse neonatal umbilical artery pH. Therefore, some of them do not recommend its use. [74, 75, 76] The study done by Paech et al [77] with subarachnoid fentanyl 20 μg+bupivacaine 2.5 mg, plus either saline or clonidine 15, 30 or 45 μg found that addition of clonidine to fentanyl-bupivacaine reduced maternal blood pressure and did not significantly augment the duration of spinal labour analgesia. To avoid hypotension due to the combination of spinal clonidine-opioids-diluted local anaesthetics, epidural clonidine can be used in doses of 75 μg. [78]

When low doses of clonidine with or without opioids are used for spinal labour analgesia, we must remember that at the end of pregnancy there is a degree of autoanalgesia mediated by endorphins [79] Even though neuraxial analgesia is the most efficient and safest mode of labour analgesia, the use of spinal clonidine mixed with opioids and/or local anaesthetics must be used cautiously to avoid hypotension.

Cesarean section. Nowadays, spinal anaesthesia is the most used technique for cesarean section. [80] Currently, opioids are the drugs most commonly used as adjuvants in this clinical scenario, but its side effects are troubling. Low doses of spinal clonidine in cesarean section are used to improve the anaesthetic block, to reduce the dose of local anaesthetics, and to prolong postoperative analgesia. It can also be combined with intrathecal opioids, as there is a synergic effect as discussed in previous paragraph.

In a recent study, 37.5 μg of clonidine added to hyperbaric bupivacaine was suggested as the optimal dose for emergency cesarean surgery, allowing reduction of up to 18% of the total dose of hyperbaric bupivacaine. [81] Adding clonidine 75μg to hyperbaric bupivacaine prolongs spinal anaesthesia and improves early postoperative analgesia after cesarean section, but does not diminish morphine needs during the first 24 hours of the postoperative period. [82] Other studies have found that 75 μg is a safe dose; prolong the anaesthetic block and enhance postoperative analgesia, with minimal side effects and no harm to the newborn. [83, 84, 85] In a randomized, double blind, dose finding study, Peach et al [86] compared intrathecal clonidine mixed with fentanyl and morphine versus clonidine plus morphine in 240 women undergoing cesarean section with hyperbaric 0.5% bupivacaine. A dose-finding analysis showed similar postoperative efficacy and side effects for groups receiving morphine 100μg with clonidine 60, 90, or 150 μg and concluded that a multimodal approach to postcesarean analgesia, using subarachnoid bupivacaine, fentanyl, morphine 100 μg, and clonidine 60 μg, improves pain relief compared with morphine 100 μg or clonidine 150 μg alone, but increases intraoperative sedation and may increase perioperative vomiting. In another dose finding study [87] comparing 15 μg, 30 μg and 60 μg of clonidine added to hyperbaric bupivacaine 0.5%, the authors found a dose dependent variability of analgesia duration and sedation. Duration of analgesia was significantly higher in those patients who received clonidine 60 μg as compared to the other two groups (598.7±140.47 versus 436.65±149.84 and 387.1±97.05 minutes respectively). Sedation was also more in the highest dose. In this study the authors recommended 15 μg and 30 μg doses due to good postoperative analgesia and less sedation.

As a single drug, subarachnoid clonidine is not recommended neither for anaesthesia or post cesarean analgesia. In order to evaluate the analgesic effect of clonidine, a double blind study was carried out in 20 patients undergoing elective cesarean section; [88] 150 μg of spinal clonidine were injected 45 min after general anaesthesia and compared to intrathecal saline as control group. Pain intensity was lower in clonidine treated patients from 20 to 120 min after intrathecal injection ($p < 0.05$), request for first analgesic was also longer in the clonidine group 414±128 min versus 181±169 min ($p < 0.01$). Clonidine side effects were severe; hypotension with a maximal reduction of systolic (15±9%), diastolic (22±12%) and mean arterial pressure

(18±12%). Sedation was significantly more intense compared to saline ($p<0.05$), also dried mouth was more commonly ($p<0.01$). Although these data suggest that 150 μg subarachnoid clonidine is effective to treat acute pain after cesarean section, it has side effects such as hypotension, sedation, and dryness of mouth.

In a research [4] using 150, 350 and 450 μg of spinal clonidine performed to evaluate the dose-response hemodynamic and analgesic profiles in the immediate postoperative period of cesarean section under general anaesthesia. The authors found that pain was less in all groups in a dose dependent mode: request for first analgesic 402±75 min, 570±76 min, and 864± 80 min respectively (p<0.01-0.001]. Clonidine reduced mean arterial pressure compared with baseline only in those patients treated with 150 μg (21±13%, $p<0.05$). Sedation was evident in all groups. Respiratory rate and motor activity of the lower extremities were unaffected in all three groups. The hemodynamic stabilility after 300 and 450 μg suggested a pressor consequence at peripheral sites. In an unpublished research we found that 75 μg of spinal clonidine was not enough to perform curettage in patients with incomplete abortion.

12. Pediatrics

Spinal anaesthesia is safe and effective in children, with many advantages like minimal cardio-respiratory disturbances. Its major limitation is its short duration, which can be extended, as in adults, with the mixture of adjuvants drugs. [90, 91] In postnatal rats, spinal clonidine did not produce signs of neurotoxicity, [33] and has been used in all pediatric age groups, from newborns to teenagers. In newborns, Rochette and coworkers [92] studied 75 patients which were injected with increasing doses of clonidine (0.25, 0.5, 1 y 2 μg/kg) with plain spinal bupivacaine 0.5% (1 mg/kg) and concluded that clonidine 1 μg/kg produces improvement in spinal anaesthesia duration without significant side effects. Dose of 2 μg/kg produced transient hypotension. In a randomized investigation with 45 children aged 6 to 15 years, clonidine 2 μg/kg prolonged motor block and improved postoperative analgesia. Hypotension and bradycardia were 54% and 30% respectively. [93] In children aged 6-8 year undergoing spinal anaesthesia with 0.5% bupivacaine for orthopedic surgery, the addition of clonidine 1 μg/kg prolonged significantly the time to regression of the sensory block and recovery of motor block, also delayed time for first rescue analgesia. Sedation was augmented and propofol requirement were reduced. [94] Batra et al [95] also demonstrated that intratecal clonidine 1 μg/kg reduces propofol dose for sedation in children.

13. Postoperative pain

The term balanced spinal analgesia refers to the antinociceptive effect produced by the interaction between several drugs that injected inside the subarachnoid space would abolish or reduce the intensity of postoperative pain. Spinal non opioids adjuvants compounds have moderate to low analgesic potency, but combined with opioids allow a decrease of opioids dose for postoperative pain control, resulting in less opioids side effects, promoting recovery and faster home readiness. Spinal alpha2 agonist drugs are not used routinely as a single analgesic in the postoperative period. A single dose of spinal clonidine as a sole postoperative analgesic has poor effect. When clonidine is added to spinal local anaesthetics or spinal opioids it does extend the time to first analgesic dose and decrease the total amount of systemic postoperative opioids. Clonidine spinal synergism with other analgesics is due to antinociceptive actions that have been described in previous paragraphs. In previous sections we have discussed some aspects of postoperative analgesia produced by intrathecal clonidine in various surgical scenarios. In this section we discuss more details on the prevention of postoperative pain with spinal clonidine.

Adding clonidine 150 μg to spinal bupivacaine in patients undergoing femoral osteosynthesis prolonged significantly the first request for analgesics compared to oral clonidine and plain spinal bupivacaine (337±29 min, 313±29 versus 236±27 min respectively), and reduced the total dose of morphine. [96] Combining 50 mg of hyperbaric lidocaine, 25 μg fentanyl, and clonidine 150 μg produced excellent postoperative analgesia in proctological patients. [97] Small doses of spinal clonidine also produce postoperative analgesia without deleterious side effects. In a comparative evaluation of 15 μg versus 30 μg clonidine as analgesic adjuvant added to 15 mg of spinal 0.5% hyperbaric bupivacaine in 90 patients undergoing abdominal hysterectomy, the authors [98] found a prolonged first pain complaint time for those women treated with clonidine compared with patients who did not received spinal clonidine (315.37+50.3, 387.07+83.19 versus 204.8+34.8 minutes). Hemodynamic parameters were alike in all patients.

A recent meta-analysis by Engelman and Marsala [99] found that clonidine increased the duration of postoperative analgesia by 1.63 h [95% confidence interval (CI): 0.93-2.33]. There was a 90% probability that clonidine increases the duration of postoperative analgesia by more than 75 min compared with morphine alone. They also found that spinal clonidine decrease the need for postoperative morphine by a mean of 4.45 mg. (95% CI: 1.40-7.49 mg). Hypotension was the only side effect increased by clonidine (odds ratio 1.78; 95% CI: 1.02-3.12). In patients undergoing transurethral surgery, 25 μg clonidine plus 7.5 mg of subarachnoid isobaric bupivacaine significantly delayed time for first request supplemental analgesia compared to bupivacaine alone (434.1±78. 3 min versus 263.97±40.38 min p=0.000) respectively. [48] In a recent study done with clonidine 30 μg added to intratecal bupivacaine-fentanyl, the authors demonstrated that the incidence of intraoperative pain and postoperative analgesic requirements were significantly less compared with the patient who did not received the alfa2 agonist for vaginal hysterectomy. [100]

Chest pain after coronary artery bypass surgery has been relieved with intrathecal clonidine in doses 1 μg/kg or 100 μg, with or without spinal opioids. Adding clonidine to neuraxial opioids improves the quality of analgesia postoperatively and expedites the process of weaning from mechanical ventilation, allowing earlier extubation. No serious side effects have been described. [101, 102, 103]

Baker and coworkers [104] hypothesized that hyperbaric clonidine avoid its rostral migration, and consequently reduced some of its side effects such as hypotension, bradycardia and sedation. They use 150 μg of either isobaric or hyperbaric clonidine in 30 elderly patients found that patients in the first group needed more intravenous fluid administration, have more bradycardia, but duration of analgesia was significantly larger than in the hyperbaric clonidine group (median, 400 min; range, 115-400 min versus median 265 min; range, 205-400 min. $p < 0.05$). Sedation scores did not differ between groups.

In conclusion, for postoperative pain the addition of clonidine to intrathecal local anaesthetics and/or opioids extends the time to first analgesia and decreases the amount of opioids used. Severe hypotension and bradycardia are seldom observed, and sedation is not an important side effect.

14. Controversy over spinal clonidine dose

As reviewed, there is no universal agreement on recommended dose for the various clinical uses of spinal clonidine. Recently, Ginosar, Riley and Angst [105] did a nice study in volunteers and found out a clonidine dose dependant effect. Significant analgesia to experimental heat pain was detected above 25 μg. After 50 μg the heat pain tolerance increased by that ~1°C, similar to the analgesic effect of 5 mg epidural morphine or 30 μg epidural fentanyl observed in studies using this experimental heat pain model.

Table 1 shows the different doses of intrathecal clonidine in different clinical scenarios of subarachnoid anaesthesia and analgesia. It can be seen that the dose range is wide as already discussed in this chapter. Up until today, there is not a standard recommended dose of subarachnoid clonidine. Doses range from 15 up to 450μg. It is necessary to adjust the dose to several factors: age, type of patients, time of surgery, type of surgery and dose of local anaesthetic and intrathecal opioids used.

Type of surgery	Dose range μg	Effects	Reported side effects	References
Ambulatory	15 to 150	Enhance anaesthesia quality	Prolongs motor block	[37, 38, 39]
		Postoperative analgesia	Hypotension	
General surgery	15 to 75	Enhance sensory and motor block	Hypotension	[41, 42, 43, 44, 45, 46]
		Decrease trans operative pain incidence	Sedation	
		Postoperative analgesia		
		Prevents postoperative hyperalgesia and chronic pain		
		Decreases postoperative analgesic consumption		
Urology	25 to 150	Shortens latency time	Bradycardia	[47, 48, 49, 50, 51]
	4 μg/kg	Retrace regression 2 segments/S1 segment	Hypotension	

Type of surgery	Dose range µg	Effects	Reported side effects	References
		Longer postoperative analgesia Reduce intraoperative opioids		
Orthopaedics	15 to 150 1-2 µg/kg	Increases regression to L1 segment and motor block duration Enhance quality anaesthesia Prolongs time for first analgesic	Facilitates high spinal block Prolongs time to void	[37, 53, 54, 55, 56, 57, 58, 60, 61]
Obstetrics				
Labour analgesia	15 to 45 50 to 200*	Potentiates opioid spinal analgesia Reduce labour pain Prolongs analgesia	Maternal hypotension Maternal dry mouth Fetal arrhythmias Fetal acidosis	[69, 70, 71, 72, 73, 74, 75, 76]
Cesarean	37.5 to 450	Enhance anaesthesia Postoperative analgesia Prolongs time for first analgesic request	Maternal hypotension Sedation	[81, 82, 83, 84, 85, 86, 87, 88]
Pediatrics	1 to 2 **	Prolongs spinal blockage Reduces propofol dose	Sedation *** Hypotension*** Respiratory depression***	[92, 93, 94, 95]
Post operative analgesia	30 to 450	Enhance spinal anaesthesia Prolongs time for first analgesic request Prolongs postoperative analgesia in a dose response manner Decrease postoperative opioids doses	Sedation Bradycardia Dose below 150 µg may induce more hypotension	[48, 96, 97, 98, 99, 100, 102, 103]

* Sole analgesic, ** µg/kg, *** Only with 2 µg/kg

Table 1. Use of spinal clonidine

15. Conclusions

Spinal anaesthesia was described over 100 years ago. Since then, neuroaxial drug administration has advanced exponentially and nowadays includes a large variety of medication that provides not only anaesthesia, but analgesia as well. The growing interest in alpha2 agonists

http://dx.doi.org/10.5772/58712

for intrathecal use has motivated innumerable research due to its ability to improve anaesthesia and neuraxial analgesia without the side effects of opioids such as respiratory depression, pruritus and urinary retention. Their analgesic effect is due to their binding on alpha2 adrenoreceptors localized in the brainstem nuclei and spinal substantia gelatinosa linked to analgesic mechanisms. A synergistic action between opioids and clonidine at the level of the spinal cord has been suggested. Clonidine also acts synergistically with local anaesthetics because of its action of opening potassium channels. Side effects of intrathecal clonidine include sedation, hypotension and a reduction of the heart rate. Spinal clonidine doses from 15 up to 450 μg are used in diverse clinical scenarios as adjuvant drug to local anaesthetics and/or opioids with the main goal to enhance spinal analgesia-anaesthesia. Clonidine and dexmedetomidine side effects are sedation, dose related bradycardia and hypotension, but rarely reach critical levels and are easy to treat. The largest evidence about the effectiveness of intrathecal clonidine is provided by studies on post-surgical pain. Although intratecal clonidine is safe, in obstetrics patients we still need to use the smallest dose based on current recommendations.

This chapter may serve as a review to help clinicians decide whether or not to use spinal clonidine as adjuvant drugs in their daily practice.

Author details

Víctor M. Whizar-Lugo[1], Juan C. Flores-Carrillo[2] and Susana Preciado-Ramírez[3]

1 Anaesthesiology, Pain Medicine, Internal Medicine and Critical Care Medicine, Hospital General de Tijuana, ISESALUD and Centro Médico del Noroeste, Tijuana , México

2 Anaesthesiology and Critical Care Medicine, Instituto Mexicano del Seguro Social and Centro Médico del Noroeste, Tijuana, México

3 Anaesthesiology Fundación Médica Sur, México D.F., México

References

[1] Bloor BC, Flacke WE. Reduction in halothane anesthetic requirement by clonidine, an alpha-adrenergic agonist. Anesth Analg 1982;61:741-5.

[2] Bloor B. Clonidine and other alpha2 adrenergic agonists: and important new drug class for the perioperative period. Sem Anesth 1988;7:170-77.

[3] Eisenach JC, De Kock M, Klimscha W.alpha(2)-adrenergic agonists for regional anesthesia. A clinical review of clonidine (1984-1995). Anesthesiology 1996;85:655-74.

[4] Filos KS, Goudas LC, Patroni O, Polyzou V. Hemodynamic and analgesic profile after intrathecal clonidine in humans. A dose-response study. Anesthesiology 1994;81:591-601.

[5] Mavropoulos G, Minguet G, Brichant JF.Interest for alpha-2 adrenoreceptor agonists in anaesthesia and intensive care medicine. Rev Med Liege 2014;69:97-101.

[6] Matsuki A. Noting new under the sun-A Japanese pioner in the clinical use of intrathecal morphine. Anesthesiology 1983;58:289-90.

[7] Yaksh TL, Rudy TA. Analgesia mediated by a direct spinal action of narcotics. Science 1976;192:1357-1358.

[8] Kroin JS, McCarthy RJ, Penn RD, Lubenow TJ, Ivankovich AD. Continuous intrathecal clonidine and tizanidine in conscious dogs: analgesic and hemodynamic effects. Anesth Analg. 2003;96:776-82.

[9] Ochs G, Loew M, Tonn J, Toyka K. Distribution, tolerability and tissue compatibility of intrathecal tizanidine in the sheep. Acta Anaesthesiol Scand 1998;42:786-93.

[10] Asano T, Dohi S, Ohta S, Shimonaka H, Iida H. Antinociception by epidural and systemic alpha(2)-adrenoceptor agonists and their binding affinity in rat spinal cord and brain. Anesth Analg. 2000;90:400-7.

[11] Stone LS, Fairbanks CA, Wilcox GL.Moxonidine, a mixed alpha(2)-adrenergic and imidazoline receptor agonist, identifies a novel adrenergic target for spinal analgesia. Ann N Y Acad Sci 2003;1009:378-85.

[12] Pettinger WA.Pharmacology of clonidine. J Cardiovasc Pharmacol 1980;2 Suppl 1:S21-8.

[13] Houston MC. Clonidine hydrochloride. South Med J 1982;75:713-9.

[14] Robinson ES, Nutt DJ, Hall L, Jackson HC, Hudson AL. Autoradiographical and behavioural effects of a chronic infusion of antisense to the alpha2D-adrenoceptor in the rat. Br J Pharmacol 1999;128:515-22.

[15] Flordellis C, Manolis A, Scheinin M, Paris H. Clinical and pharmacological significance of alpha2-adrenoceptor polymorphisms in cardiovascular diseases. Int J Cardiol 2004;97:367-72.

[16] Odagaki Y, Toyoshima R.Pharmacological characterization of alpha2D-adrenergic receptor-mediated [35S]GTPgammaS binding in rat cerebral cortical membranes. Pharmacol Res 2008;57:435-44.

[17] Quaglia W, Del Bello F, Giannella M, Piergentili A, Pigini M. α2C-adrenoceptor modulators: a patent review. Expert Opin Ther Pat 2011;21:455-81.

[18] Civantos Calzada B, Aleixandre de Artiñano A. Alpha-adrenoceptor subtypes. Pharmacol Res 2001;44:195-208.

http://dx.doi.org/10.5772/58712

[19] Lee A, Rosin DL, Van Bockstaele EJ.Ultrastructural evidence for prominent postsynaptic localization of alpha2C-adrenergic receptors in catecholaminergic dendrites in the rat nucleus locus coeruleus. J Comp Neurol 1998;394:218-29.

[20] Pan HL, Wu ZZ, Zhou HY, et al. Modulation of pain transmission by G-protein-coupled receptors. Pharmacol Ther 2008;117:141-61.

[21] Valenzuela-Harrington M, Negrete-Díaz V, Rodríguez-Moreno A. Núcleo coeruleous. Neurotrasmisores, funciones y patología. Anest Mex 2007:19;155-66.

[22] Whizar-Lugo V. El núcleo coeruleus, receptores alfa2 adrenérgicos y anestesia. Anest Mex 2007;19:130-34.

[23] Wei ZY, Karim F, Roerig SC. Spinal morphine/clonidine antinociceptive synergism: involvement of G proteins and N-type voltage-dependent calcium channels. J Pharmacol Exp Ther 1996;278:1392-407.

[24] Wilcox GL, Carlsson KH, Jochim A, Jurna I. Mutual potentiation of antinociceptive effects of morphine and clonidine on motor and sensory responses in rat spinal cord. Brain Res 1987;405:84-93.

[25] Roerig SC, Lei S, Kitto K, Hylden JK, Wilcox GL. Spinal interactions between opioid and noradrenergic agonists in mice: multiplicativity involves delta and alpha-2 receptors. J Pharmacol Exp Ther. 1992;262:365-74.

[26] Stone LS, MacMillan LB, Kitto KF, Limbird LE, Wilcox GL. The alpha2a adrenergic receptor subtype mediates spinal analgesia evoked by alpha2 agonists and is necessary for spinal adrenergic-opioid synergy. J Neurosci. 1997;17:7157-65.

[27] Fairbanks CA, Stone LS, Kitto KF, et al.alpha(2C)-Adrenergic receptors mediate spinal analgesia and adrenergic-opioid synergy. J Pharmacol Exp Ther 2002;300:282-90.

[28] Chabot-Doré AJ, Millecamps M, Stone LS. The delta-opioid receptor is sufficient, but not necessary, for spinal opioid-adrenergic analgesic synergy. J Pharmacol Exp Ther 2013;347:773-80.

[29] Schuster DJ, Kitto KF, Overland AC, et al.Protein kinase Cε is required for spinal analgesic synergy between delta opioid and alpha-2A adrenergic receptor agonist pairs. J Neurosci. 2013;33:13538-46.

[30] Guevara-López U, Aldrete JA, Covarrubias-Gómez A, Hernández-Pando RE, López-Muñoz FJ. Absence of histological changes after the administration of a continuous intrathecal clonidine in Wistar rats. Pain Pract. 2009;9:122-9.

[31] Erdivanli B, Altun M, Sezen OK, Colakoğlu SA. Anti-nociceptive, analgesic and pathohistological effects of intrathecal dexmedetomidine and bupivacaine in rats. Rev Bras Anestesiol. 2013;63:183-7.

[32] Zhang H, Zhou F, Li C, et al. Molecular mechanisms underlying the analgesic property of intrathecal dexmedetomidine and its neurotoxicity evaluation: an in vivo and in vitro experimental study. PLoS One. 2013;8:e55556.

[33] Walker SM, Grafe M, Yaksh TL Intratecal clonidine in the neonatal rat: Dose-dependent analgesia and evaluation of spinal apoptosis toxicity. Anesth Analg 2012:115;450-460.

[34] Elia N, Culebras X, Mazza C, Schiffer E, Tramèr MR. Clonidine as an adjuvant to intrathecal local anesthetics for surgery: systematic review of randomized trials. Reg Anesth Pain Med. 2008;33:159-67.

[35] Whizar-Lugo VM, Martínez-Gallegos N, Torres-Chávez J. Polémicas en anestesia subaracnoidea. Anest Mex 2004;16:109-123.

[36] Salinas FV, Liu SS.Spinal anaesthesia: local anaesthetics and adjuncts in the ambulatory setting. Best Pract Res Clin Anaesthesiol. 2002;16:195-210.

[37] van Tuijl I, Giezeman MJ, Braithwaite SA, Hennis PJ, Kalkman CJ, van Klei WA.Intrathecal low-dose hyperbaric bupivacaine-clonidine combination in outpatient knee arthroscopy: a randomized controlled trial. Acta Anaesthesiol Scand 2008;52:343-9.

[38] Merivirta R, Kuusniemi K, Jaakkola P, Pihlajamäki K, Pitkänen M. Unilateral spinal anaesthesia for outpatient surgery: a comparison between hyperbaric bupivacaine and bupivacaine-clonidine combination. Acta Anaesthesiol Scand. 2009;53:788-93.

[39] De Kock M, Gautier P, Fanard L, Hody JL, Lavand'homme P. Intrathecal ropivacaine and clonidine for ambulatory knee arthroscopy: a dose-response study. Anesthesiology 2001;94:574-8.

[40] Julião MC, Lauretti GR.Low-dose intrathecal clonidine combined with sufentanil as analgesic drugs in abdominal gynecological surgery. J Clin Anesth. 2000;12:357-62.

[41] Braz JR, Koguti ES, Braz LG, Croitor LB, Navarro LH. Effects of clonidine associated to hyperbaric bupivacaine during high-level spinal anesthesia. Rev Bras Anestesiol 2003;53:561-72.

[42] Yoganarasimha N, Raghavendra T, Amitha S, Shridhar K, Radha M. A comparative study between intrathecal clonidine and neostigmine with intrathecal bupivacaine for lower abdominal surgeries. Indian J Anaesth. 2014;58:43-7.

[43] De Kock M, Lavand'homme P, Waterloos H.The short-lasting analgesia and long-term antihyperalgesic effect of intrathecal clonidine in patients undergoing colonic surgery. Anesth Analg 2005;101:566-72.

[44] Ghodki PS, Sardesai SP, Thombre SK.Evaluation of the effect of intrathecal clonidine to decrease shoulder tip pain in laparoscopy under spinal anaesthesia. Indian J Anaesth 2010;54:231-4.

[45] Dobrydnjov I, Axelsson K, Thörn SE, et al. Clonidine combined with small-dose bupivacaine during spinal anesthesia for inguinal herniorrhaphy: a randomized double-blinded study. Anesth Analg 2003;96:1496-503.

[46] Thakur A, Bhardwaj M, Kaur K, et al. Intrathecal clonidine as an adjuvant to hyperbaric bupivacaine in patients undergoing inguinal herniorrhaphy: A randomized double-blinded study. J Anaesthesiol Clin Pharmacol 2013;29:66-70.

[47] Santiveri X, Arxer A, Plaja I, Metje MT, Martínez B, Villalonga A, López M. Anaesthetic and postoperative analgesic effects of spinal clonidine as an additive to prilocaine in the transurethral resection of urinary bladder tumours. Eur J Anaesthesiol 2002;19:589-93.

[48] Gecaj-Gashi A, Terziqi H, Pervorfi T, Kryeziu A. Intrathecal clonidine added to small-dose bupivacaine prolongs postoperative analgesia in patients undergoing transurethral surgery. Can Urol Assoc J 2012;6:25-9.

[49] Kanazi GE, Aouad MT, Jabbour-Khoury SI, et al.. Effect of low-dose dexmedetomidine or clonidine on the characteristics of bupivacaine spinal block. Acta Anaesthesiol Scand 2006;50:222-7.

[50] Andrieu G, Roth B, Ousmane L, et al. The efficacy of intrathecal morphine with or without clonidine for postoperative analgesia after radical prostatectomy. Anesth Analg 2009;108:1954-7.

[51] Larsen B, Dorscheid E, Macher-Hanselmann F, Büch U. Does intrathecal clonidine prolong the effect of spinal anesthesia with hyperbaric mepivacaine? A randomized double-blind study. Anaesthesist 1998;47:741-6.

[52] Ouro-Bang'na Maman AF, Sama HD, Alassani F, Egbohou P, Chobli M. Severe differed respiratory depression after intrathecal administration of morphine and clonidine on a 70-year-old patient. Ann Fr Anesth Reanim 2009;28:701-3.

[53] Strebel S, Gurzeler JA, Schneider MC, Aeschbach A, Kindler CH. Small-dose intrathecal clonidine and isobaric bupivacaine for orthopedic surgery: a dose-response study. Anesth Analg 2004;99:1231-8.

[54] Amaranto MA, Berrío C. Clonidina por vía subaracnoidea en pacientes de traumatología. Rev Colomb Anestesiol 2000;28:149-56.

[55] Kaabachi O, Zarghouni A, Ouezini R, Abdelaziz AB, Chattaoui O, Kokki H. Clonidine 1 microg/kg is a safe and effective adjuvant to plain bupivacaine in spinal anesthesia in adolescents. Anesth Analg. 2007;105:516-9.

[56] Fournier R, Van Gessel E, Weber A, Gamulin Z. Epinephrine and clonidine do not improve intrathecal sufentanil analgesia after total hip replacement. Br J Anaesth 2002;89:562-6.

[57] Mahendru V, Tewari A, Katyal S, et al. A comparison of intrathecal dexmedetomidine, clonidine, and fentanyl as adjuvants to hyperbaric bupivacaine for lower limb

surgery: A double blind controlled study. J Anaesthesiol Clin Pharmacol. 2013;29:496-502.

[58] Agarwal D, Chopra M, Mohta M, Sethi AK. Clonidine as an adjuvant to hyperbaric bupivacaine for spinal anesthesia in elderly patients undergoing lower limb orthopedic surgeries. Saudi J Anaesth 2014;8:209-14.

[59] Dobrydnjov I, Axelsson K, Gupta A, et al. Improved analgesia with clonidine when added to local anesthetic during combined spinal-epidural anesthesia for hip arthroplasty: a double-blind, randomized and placebo-controlled study. Acta Anaesthesiol Scand 2005;49:538-45.

[60] Gehling M, Tryba M, Lüsebrink T, Zorn A. Can the addition of clonidine improve the analgesic efficacy of low dose intrathecal morphine? A randomised double-blind trial. Anaesthesist 2003;52:204-9.

[61] Grace D, Milligan KR, Morrow BJ, Fee JP. Co-administration of pethidine and clonidine: a spinal anaesthetic technique for total hip replacement. Br J Anaesth 1994;73:628-33.

[62] Hong RW. Less is more: the recent history of neuraxial labor analgesia. Am J Ther. 2010;17:492-7.

[63] Roelants F. The use of neuraxial adjuvant drugs (neostigmine, clonidine) in obstetrics. Curr Opin Anaesthesiol 2006;19:233-7.

[64] Datta S. Spinal opiates in obstetrics. In Obstetric anaesthesia handbook. Fourth Edition. Springer USA. Pags 89-99. 2006.

[65] Goudra BG, Singh PM. Remifentanil in labor. J Obstet Anaesth Crit Care 2013;3:74-6.

[66] Sultan P, Murphy C, Halpern S, Carvalho B. The effect of low concentrations versus high concentrations of local anesthetics for labour analgesia on obstetric and anesthetic outcomes: a meta-analysis. Can J Anaesth 2013;60:840-54.

[67] Pandya ST. Labour analgesia: Recent advances. Indian J Anaesth. 2010;54:400-8.

[68] Van de Velde M. Neuraxial analgesia and fetal bradycardia. Curr Opin Anaesthesiol 2005;18:253-6.

[69] Mercier FJ, Boulay G, Ben Ayed M, Benhamou D.Combined spinal and epidural analgesia for labor. Prolongation by addition of a minidose of clonidine to sufentanil. An initial study. Ann Fr Anesth Reanim 1996;15:263-5.

[70] Mercier FJ, Dounas M, Bouaziz H, Des Mesnards-Smaja V, Foiret C, Vestermann MN, Fischler M, Benhamou D. The effect of adding a minidose of clonidine to intrathecal sufentanil for labor analgesia. Anesthesiology 1998;89:594-601.

[71] Gautier PE, De Kock M, Fanard L, Van Steenberge A, Hody JL. Intrathecal clonidine combined with sufentanil for labor analgesia. Anesthesiology 1998;88:651-6.

[72] Labbene I, Gharsallah H, Abderrahman A, et al. Effects of 15 mcg intrathecal clonidine added to bupivacaine and sufentanil for labor analgesia.Tunis Med 2011;89:853-9.

[73] Chiari A, Lorber C, Eisenach JC, et al. Analgesic and hemodynamic effects of intrathecal clonidine as the sole analgesic agent during first stage of labor: a dose-response study. Anesthesiology 1999;91:388-96.

[74] Missant C, Teunkens A, Vandermeersch E, Van de Velde M. Intrathecal clonidine prolongs labour analgesia but worsens fetal outcome: a pilot study. Can J Anaesth. 2004;51:696-701.

[75] Dewandre PY. The right drug and dose for neuraxial labour analgesia. Acta Anaesthesiol Belg 2006;57:395-9.

[76] Belhadj Amor M1, Draief A, Ouezini R, Dhahri S, Jebali A, Lamine K, Ferjani M. 30 microg intrathecal clonidine prolongs labour analgesia, but increases the incidence of hypotension and abnormal foetal heart rate patterns. Ann Fr Anesth Reanim. 2007;26:916-20.

[77] Paech MJ, Banks SL, Gurrin LC, Yeo ST, Pavy TJ. A randomized, double-blinded trial of subarachnoid bupivacaine and fentanyl, with or without clonidine, for combined spinal/epidural analgesia during labor. Anesth Analg 2002;95:1396-401.

[78] Van de Velde M, Berends N, Kumar A, Devroe S, Devlieger R, Vandermeersch E, De Buck F.Effects of epidural clonidine and neostigmine following intrathecal labour analgesia: a randomised, double-blind, placebo-controlled trial. Int J Obstet Anesth. 2009;18:207-14.

[79] Eisenach JC, Dobson CE, Inturissi CE, Hood D, Agner PB. Effect of pregnancy and pain on cerebrospinal fluid immunoreactive enkephalins and norepinephrine in healthy humans Pain 1990;43:149-54.

[80] Arzola C, Wieczorek PM. Efficacy of low-dose bupivacaine in spinal anaesthesia for Caesarean delivery: systematic review and meta-analysis. Br J Anaesth 2011;107:308-18.

[81] Bajwa SJ, Bajwa SK, Kaur J, Singh A, Singh A, Parmar SS. Prevention of hypotension and prolongation of postoperative analgesia in emergency cesarean sections: A randomized study with intrathecal clonidine. Int J Crit Illn Inj Sci 2012;2:63-9.

[82] van Tuijl I, van Klei WA, van der Werff DB, Kalkman CJ. The effect of addition of intrathecal clonidine to hyperbaric bupivacaine on postoperative pain and morphine requirements after Caesarean section: a randomized controlled trial. Br J Anaesth 2006;97:365-70.

[83] Bhure A, Kalita N, Ingley P, Gadkari CP. Comparison of different doses of clonidine as an adjuvant to intrathecal bupivacaine for spinal anesthesia and postoperative an-

algesia in patients undergoing caesarian section. People's Journal of Scientific Research 2012;5:19-23.

[84] Marzieh Beigom Khezri, Meisam Rezaei, Morteza Delkhosh Reihany, Ezzatalsadat Haji Seid Javadi. Comparison of postoperative analgesic effect of intrathecal clonidine and fentanyl added to bupivacaine in patients undergoing cesarean section: A prospective randomized double-blind study. Pain Res Treat 2014; Article ID 513628, 7 pages.

[85] Singh R, Gupta D, Jain A.The effect of addition of intrathecal clonidine to hyperbaric bupivacaine on postoperative pain after lower segment caesarean section: A randomized control trial. Saudi J Anaesth 2013;7:283-90.

[86] Paech MJ, Pavy TJ, Orlikowski CE, Yeo ST, Banks SL, Evans SF, Henderson J. Postcesarean analgesia with spinal morphine, clonidine, or their combination. Anesth Analg 2004;98:1460-6.

[87] Shah BB, Joshi SS, Shidhaye RV, Lakhe JN. Comparison of different doses of clonidine as an adjuvant to intrathecal bupivacaine for spinal anesthesia and postoperative analgesia in patients undergoing caesarian section. Anaesth Pain & Intensive Care 2012;16:266-72.

[88] Filos KS, Goudas LC, Patroni O, Polyzou V. Intrathecal clonidine as a sole analgesic for pain relief after cesarean section. Anesthesiology 1992;77:267-74.

[89] Polati E, Finco G, Bartoloni A, et al. Treatment of postoperative pain by balanced spinal analgesia. Chir Ital 1995;47:30-6.

[90] Kokki H. Spinal blocks. Paediatr Anaesth. 2012;22:56-64.

[91] Gupta A, Saha U. Spinal anesthesia in children: A review. J Anaesthesiol Clin Pharmacol 2014;30:10-18.

[92] Rochette A, Raux O, Troncin R, et al.. Clonidine prolongs spinal anesthesia in newborns: a prospective dose-ranging study. Anesth Analg 2004;98:56-9.

[93] Kaabachi O, Ben Rajeb A, Mebazaa M, Safi H, Jelel C, Ben Ghachem M, Ben Ammar M. Spinal anesthesia in children: comparative study of hyperbaric bupivacaine with or without clonidine. Ann Fr Anesth Reanim 2002;21:617-21.

[94] Cao JP, Miao XY, Liu J, Shi XY. An evaluation of intrathecal bupivacaine combined with intrathecal or intravenous clonidine in children undergoing orthopedic surgery: a randomized double-blinded study. Paediatr Anaesth 2011;21:399-405.

[95] Batra YK, Rakesh SV, Panda NB, Lokesh VC, Subramanyam R. Intrathecal clonidine decreases propofol sedation requirements during spinal anesthesia in infants. Paediatr Anaesth 2010;20:625-32.

[96] Dobrydnjov I, Axelsson K, Samarütel J, Holmström B.Postoperative pain relief following intrathecal bupivacaine combined with intrathecal or oral clonidine. Acta Anaesthesiol Scand. 2002;46:806-14.

[97] Martínez GL, Alfonso R. León V AR, Orizondo PS. Clonidina intratecal para alivio del dolor posoperatorio en cirugía proctológica. Su combinación con otros agentes. Rev Cubana Cir 2001;40:297-304.

[98] Singh YA, Dwivedib S, Yadav K. Comparative evaluation of effects of different doses of intrathecal clonidine with bupivacaine on post operative pain relief. Int J Biol Med Res 2013; 4:2703-06.

[99] Engelman E, Marsala C. Efficacy of adding clonidine to intrathecal morphine in acute postoperative pain: meta-analysis. Br J Anaesth 2013;110:21-7.

[100] Chopra P, Talwar V. Low dose intrathecal clonidine and fentanyl added to hyperbaric bupivacaine prolongs analgesia in gynecological surgery. J Anaesthesiol Clin Pharmacol 2014;30:233-7.

[101] Nader ND, Li CM, Dosluoglu HH, Ignatowski TA, Spengler RN. Adjuvant therapy with intrathecal clonidine improves postoperative pain in patients undergoing coronary artery bypass graft. Clin J Pain 2009;25:101-6.

[102] Lena P, Balarac N, Arnulf JJ, Teboul J, Bonnet F. Intrathecal morphine and clonidine for coronary artery bypass grafting. Br J Anaesth 2003;90:300-3.

[103] Lena P, Balarac N, Arnulf JJ, et al.. Fast-track coronary artery bypass grafting surgery under general anesthesia with remifentanil and spinal analgesia with morphine and clonidine. J Cardiothorac Vasc Anesth. 2005;19:49-53.

[104] Baker A, Klimscha W, Eisenach JC, et al. Intrathecal clonidine for postoperative analgesia in elderly patients: the influence of baricity on hemodynamic and analgesic effects. Anesth Analg 2004;99:128-34.

[105] Ginosar Y, Riley ET, Angst MS. Analgesic and sympatholytic effects of low-dose intrathecal clonidine compared with bupivacaine: a dose-response study in female volunteers. Br J Anaesth 2013;111:256-63.

Chapter 6

Midazolam in Spinal Anesthesia — Intrathecal or Intravenous?

Beyazit Zencirci

Additional information is available at the end of the chapter

http://dx.doi.org/10.5772/58750

1. Introduction

The first spinal anesthesia was carried out by Dr August Bier in 1899 and his anesthetic technique has become the standard practice for lower extremity and abdominal surgery worldwide [1]. Nowadays, the most commonly used drugs for spinal anesthesia are local anesthetics. However, a major disadvantage of single injection spinal anesthesia is its limited duration of action. In clinical practice, a number of adjuvants have been added to intrathecal local anesthetics for supplementation of intraoperative anesthesia and postoperative analgesia. They have advantages as they reduce the dose of local anesthetic; provide long lasting postoperative analgesia with reduced incidence of central nervous system depression, motor effects or hypotension [2].

Midazolam, synthesized by Walsar and colleagues in 1976, was the first clinically used water soluble benzodiazepine [3]. It is also the first benzodiazepine that was produced primarily for use in anesthesia [4]. In 1986, Faull and Villiger demonstrated that there is a high density of benzodiazepine (*GABA-A*) receptors in lamina II of the dorsal horn in the human spinal cord, suggesting a possible role in pain modulation [5]. One year later, Goodchild and Serrao reported that benzodiazepines might have analgesic effects at the spinal cord level in animals [6]. In 1990s, analgesic efficacy of intrathecal midazolam in humans has been demonstrated [7-9]. Naltrindole, a δ-selective opioid antagonistic agent, suppresses the antinociceptive effect of intrathecal midazolam, suggesting that intrathecal midazolam is involved in the release of an endogenous opioid acting at spinal δ receptors [10].

This chapter is going to focus on the relationship between midazolam and spinal anesthesia.

2. Midazolam

Benzodiazepines commonly used in the perioperative period include diazepam, midazolam, and lorazepam, as well as the selective benzodiazepine antagonist flumazenil (Figure 1). The chemical structure of the benzodiazepines contains a benzene ring fused to a seven-member diazepine ring, hence their name. They are all composed of a benzene ring (*A*) fused to a seven-membered 1, 4-diazepine ring (*B*). Anesthesiologically relevant benzodiazepine agonists also contain a 5-aryl substituent (*ring* C), which enhances the pharmacological potency. However, the benzodiazepine antagonist flumazenil has two important structural differences as compared to the above agonists. Flumazenil has a keto function at position 5 instead of ring C, and a methyl substituent at position 4. Hence benzodiazepines are unique among the group of intravenous anesthetics in that their action can readily be terminated by administration of their selective antagonist flumazenil [11, 12].

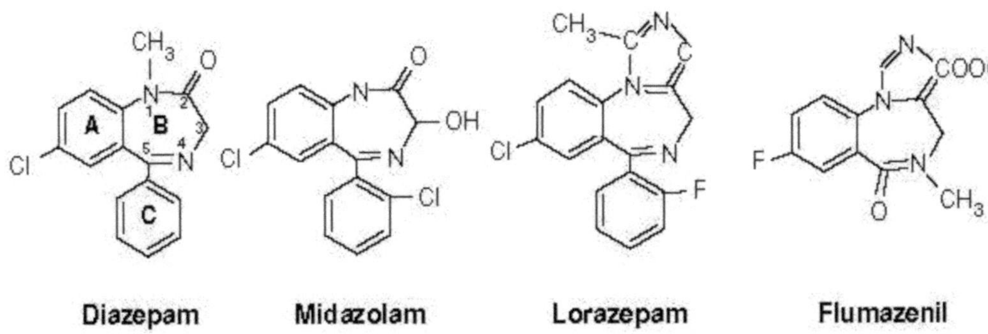

Figure 1. Chemical structure of the three commonly used benzodiazepines and their antogonist flumazenil.

Midazolam is an imidazobenzodiazepine. This results in the ability of a water molecule to open the diazepine ring, thus encouraging aqueous solubility. The equilibrium between the two forms of midazolam is determined by pH. The change from one form to the other is relatively slow, having a half-life of 10 minutes. The pH in the ampoule containing midazolam hydrochloride is 3.0 and so the ring is open and it is soluble. Once subjected to body pH 7.4, the diazepine ring closes and the midazolam becomes lipid-soluble, allowing it readily to cross the blood–brain barrier. In the plasma most of the midazolam (95%) is protein-bound. Small changes in its plasma protein binding will produce large changes in the amount of free drug available, which may have consequences in clinical practice [13]. The high lipophilicity of midazolam accounts for the relatively large volume of distribution at steady-state [14]. Older age does not increase the volume of distribution significantly [15, 16]. However, in obese patients, the volume of distribution is increased and the elimination half-time is prolonged while the clearance remains unchanged [15].

Elimination half-time is independent of the route of administration. Major operations seem to increase the volume of distribution and prolong the elimination half-time [16]. Following intravenous administration, midazolam is rapidly distributed and the distribution half-time is 6-15 min [17]. The fused imidazole ring of midazolam is oxidized much more rapidly than the methylene group of the diazepine ring of other benzodiazepines [18-20]. In elderly men, the clearance of midazolam is reduced and the elimination half-time is prolonged as compared to young males. Between elderly and young women, however, no significant differences were detected in the clearance or the elimination halftime of midazolam [15]. In addition to the liver, midazolam is also metabolized at extrahepatic sites. This has been demonstrated by the discovery of metabolites following intravenous injection of midazolam during the anhepatic period of liver transplantation [21]. In patients with advanced cirrhosis of the liver, the plasma clearance is reduced and the elimination half-time is prolonged as compared to healthy volunteers, while the volume of distribution remains unchanged [22].

The first step in the metabolism of midazolam is hydroxylation [23]. The two metabolites formed are α-hydroxymidazolam and 4-hydroxymidazolam, both are pharmacologically active [14, 24]. The α-hydroxymidazolam is as potent as the parent compound and may contribute significantly to the effects of the parent drug when present in sufficiently high concentrations. 4-Hydroxymidazolam is quantitatively unimportant [25]. Both metabolites are rapidly conjugated by glucuronic acid to form products which have been considered to be pharmacologically inactive [14]. On the other hand; glucuronidated α-hydroxymidazolam, the main metabolite of midazolam, has a substantial pharmacological effect and can penetrate the intact blood–brain barrier. The elimination half-time of α-hydroxymidazolam is about 70 min [25]. However, it can accumulate in patients with renal failure. Furthermore, in vitro binding studies show that the affinity of glucuronidated α-hydroxymidazolam to the cerebral benzodiazepine receptor is only about ten times weaker than that of midazolam or unconjugated α-hydroxymidazolam [26].

Midazolam is supplied as hydrochloride salt with a pH less than 4.0 (*buffered to an acidic pH of 3.5*). This is important because midazolam displays pH-dependent solubility. The diazepine ring of midazolam accounts for its stability in solution and rapid metabolism. It remains open at pH value of <4, thus maintaining drug´s water solubility. The ring closes at pH value of > 4, as when the drug is exposed to physiologic pH, thus converting midazolam to a highly lipid soluble drug [27] and this lipophilicity is responsible for its rapid CNS effect and large volume of distribution [28]. Therefore the pH of the commercial midazolam hydrochloride preparation is adjusted to 3 with hydrochloride acid and sodium hydroxide. As midazolam is injected into patients, pH is increased and the ring is closed thus increasing the lipid solubility.

Midazolam exerts its effect by occupying benzodiazepine receptor that modulates γ-amino butyric acid (*GABA*), the major inhibitory neurotransmitter in the brain. Benzodiazepine receptors are found in the olfactory bulb, cerebral cortex, cerebellum, hippocampus, substantia nigra, inferior colliculus, brain stem, and spinal cord. There are two types of GABA receptors; benzodiazepine receptors are part of the benzodiazepine-GABAA-chloride channel receptor complex. Benzodiazepine binding site is located on the γ2 subunit of the GABA receptor complex [29, 30]. With the activation of the GABAA receptor, gating of the channel for chloride ions is started after which the cell becomes hyperpolarised and resistant to neuronal excitation. The hypnotic effects of benzodiazepine are mediated by alterations in the potential dependent calcium ion flux [31]. Hypnotic, sedative, amnesic, and anticonvulsant effects are mediated by

$\alpha 1$ GABA receptors and anxiolysis and centrally acting muscle relexant properties are mediated by $\alpha 2$ GABA receptors [31].

The anxiolytic effect of midazolam is via its action at mammillary body. Presumably midazolam exerts its anxiolytic property like other benzodiazepines by increasing glycine inhibitory neurotransmitter. Midazolam also possesses anticonvulsant action which is attributed to enhanced activity of GABA on the brain's motor circuit. It exhibits a muscle relaxant effect via its action at the glycine receptors in the spinal cord. Midazolam administered via intrathecal or epidural routes can produce analgesia, probably due to its GABA mediated action [4]. Other mechanisms of action including its interaction with opiate receptors have also been proposed [10].

3. Intrathecal midazolam: Useful or toxic?

Spinal anesthesia is the most commonly used regional anesthetic technique. Local anesthetic agents used for this purpose provide good intraoperative analgesia. However, they provide a very limited postoperative duration of action. In order to overcome this problem and to maximise the duration of anesthesia-analgesia, many adjuvants, such as intrathecal opioids and non-opioids, have increasingly been tried in the last two decades to relieve postoperative pain [32-34]. Among the various methods availabe for providing post-operative analgesia, the benefits of intrathecal opioids and non-opioids as adjuncts in spinal anaesthesia are well documented. Unfortunately the addition of intrathecal opioids is associated with dose-related adverse effects such as respiratory depression, nausea, vomiting, urinary retention, pruritus, and sedation [35]. Therefore, the use of non-opioids such as ketamine, clonidine, neostigmine, magnesium sulfate, and midazolam have become popular adjuncts for post-operative analgesia. However, side-effects in the postoperative period render most adjuvants less than ideal.

Midazolam, a water soluble benzodiazepine, has been used via intrathecal route in the management of acute (*perioperative*) [36, 37], chronic [38] and cancer [39] pain. Goodchild and Noble were the first to demonstrate the role of intrathecal midazolam in relieving pain of somatic origin in humans [36]. The rationale for the use of intrathecal midazolam focuses on the awareness that it is an agonist at the benzodiazepine binding site, a subunit of the pentameric gammaaminobutyric acid (*GABA-A*) receptor. Agonist occupancy of the benzodiazepine binding site enhances the activity of GABA at the GABA-A receptor. The GABA receptor is a chloride ionophore that, when activated, typically stabilises the transmembrane potential at, or near, the resting potential. In neurons, this typically serves to decrease excitability [40]. Intrathecal benzodiazepine-induced analgesia is spinally mediated. Binding sites are GABA receptors, abundantly present in the dorsal root nerve cells, with the maximum concentration found within lamina II of the dorsal nerve cells, a region that plays a prominent role in processing nociceptive and thermoceptive stimulation [36]. The present cumulative experience with intrathecal midazolam across species broadly confirms the safety thereof, the analgesic activity of the molecule and its benzodiazepine pharmacology, and the lack of irreversible effects [8].

Intrathecal midazolam was originally shown to have antinociceptive properties in animals in the early 1980s [41, 42]. And later in 1991, Malinovsky et al. demonstrated potential of neurotoxic effect of intrathecal administration of ketamine and midazolam in rabbits [43]. Midazolam-treated rabbits showed significant changes in both blood-brain barrier and light microscopy studies. They postulated that, the neurotoxicity might be due to the 10% HCL used as a vehicle in the preparation of midazolam. In 1999 Erdine et al. conducted a study of intrathecal midazolam in rabbits and reported neurotoxicity [44]. They concluded that the neurotoxicity was due to the use of intrathecal catheter. They also reported that this toxic change did not produce any change in the vital parameters of those animals. However, in 1991 Schoeffler et al. conducted a detailed histological study in rats following administration of midazolam via subarachnoid catheter while investigating control of cancer pain [45]. They found that the amount of fibrosis, infiltration, and deformation in midazolam group is not different from saline control group. Aguilar et al. in 1994, conducted study and reported that intrathecal midazolam can relieve pain in different clinical situations (*as long as 13 months*) and they did not show any toxic neurological effects following prolonged administration of intrathecal midazolam [46]. Nevetheless, in 1995 Svensson et al. conducted a morphological study on rat spinal cords following chronic subarachnoid administration of midazolam, documenting its neurotoxic effect [47].

In 1996, Valentine et al. studied the effect of intrathecal midazolam along with hyperbaric bupivacaine for caesarean section delivery under spinal anaesthesia and found no side effects attributable to midazolam [8]. In the same year, Borg and Krijnen reported long-term intrathecal administration of midazolam and clonidine in patients with refractory musculoskeletal pain persisting more than 2.5 years [9]. They administered intrathecal midazolam up to 6mg/day which showed promising results, they also reported that this high dose did not cause any neurological deficits in those patients suffering with chronic refractory musculoskeletal pain [9]. One year later, Bozkurt et al. studied the histological change following epidural administration of midazolam in neonatal rabbits and showed a variable degree of neurotoxic effects such as degeneration of vacuoles, cytoplasm and neurofilaments, disruption of myelin sheaths, lysis of cell membranes, perivascular oedema, and pyknosis of nuclei [48]. The toxic effects of acidic saline and midazolam (*commercially available preparations*) were similar. In the same year, Bahar et al. examined in an animal model whether intrathecal midazolam, alone or with fentanyl, can achieve anaesthesia sufficient for laparotomy, comparable to lidocaine; they concluded that midazolam, when injected intrathecally, produces reversible, segmental, spinally mediated antinociception, sufficient to provide balanced anaesthesia without any adverse effect [49]. In 1999, Nishiyama et al. conducted histopathological study in cats with intrathecal midazolam. Neither acute histological damage nor inflammatory reaction of the spinal cord were seen in the cats [50].

In 1998, Nishiyama et al. studied the effect of continuous infusion of midazolam with local anesthetic for treatment of postoperative pain and showed that adding midazolam to a continuous epidural infusion of bupivacaine provides better analgesia, amnesia, and sedation than bupivacaine alone without any side effects [51]. Also Nishiyama et al. in the same year studied the effect of adding midazolam and bupivacaine to human cerebrospinal fluid in glass test tubes and the solution was examined for any change of pH and a reduction in the transparency of the solution [52]. Cerebrospinal pH was decreased to below 7.0 adding more than 3 mg of midazolam, more than 1.9 mL of 0.25% bupivacaine or 1.3 mL of the mixture. Cerebrospinal transparency by adding more than 0.7 mg of midazolam, 1.1 mL of 0.25% bupivacaine or 0.6 mL of the mixture. Midazolam in saline neither decreased the pH below nor reduced transparency. These results are very important so this study showed that clinically useful doses of intrathecal or epidural midazolam were not neurotoxic. In the same year, Gulec et al. showed that caudal administration of a bupivacaine-midazolam mixture produces a longer duration of postoperative analgesia than a bupivacaine-morphine mixture and bupivacaine alone [53]. Batra et al. in 1999, conducted a study on postoperative analgesia in patients undergoing knee arthroscopy following intrathecal administration of midazolam in combination with hyperbaric bupivacaine [54]. They demonstrated that this combination produces better postoperative analgesia. In 2001, Kim and Lee showed a dose-dependent effect of intrathecal midazolam [55]. Sen et al. reported that intrathecal midazolam produced significant postoperative pain relief together with antiemetic effect and tranquillity in patients undergoing caesarean section delivery [56]. Maharjan et al showed that caudal administration of midazolam-bupivacaine mixture significantly prolongs postoperative analgesia compared to bupivacaine alone in children undergoing genitourinary surgery [57]. Moreover, other studies have shown that addition of intrathecal midazolam significantly improves the duration and quality of spinal anesthesia and provides prolonged perioperative analgesia without any significant side effects and neurological damage [58-61]. Prochazka shared their decade long experience of using intrathecal midazolam in 2006 [62]. According to them, intrathecal midazolam is able to provide good analgesia in most patients and is a very suitable supplement for postoperative and long-term analgesia without demand of expensive systems (*Patient Controlled Analgesia and other drug infusion systems, etc.*). On the other hand, recent studies showed that intrathecal midazolam appears to improve perioperative analgesia and it can be useful and safe adjunct to bupivacaine for intrathecal analgesia during different surgical operations [35, 63-66].

Yegin et al. in 2004, conducted a study on the analgesic and sedative effects of intrathecal 2mg preservative free midazolam in perianal surgery under spinal anesthesia [37]. They found that the addition of bupivacaine produces a more effective and longer analgesia with a mild sedative effect in patients in the experimental group. One year later Agrawal et al. investigated postoperative pain relief following intrathecal administration of 1mg preservative free midazolam with bupivacaine in patients scheduled for elective lower abdominal, lower limb, and endoscopic urological surgeries [67]. They showed that intrathecal midazolam and bupivacaine provide longer duration of postoperative analgesia as compared to intrathecal bupivacaine alone, without prolonging time for dermatomal regression. Also, Prakash et al. [35] with Ho and Ismail [64] found that intrathecal midazolam appears to improve perioperative analgesia and reduce nausea and vomiting during caesarean delivery. On the other hand in 2011, Shadangi et al. concluded that the addition of preservative-free midazolam to bupivacaine intrathecally resulted in prolonged postoperative analgesia without increasing motor block [68].

Addition of preservative free midazolam to hyperbaric bupivacaine for spinal anesthesia in different surgical procedures/operations prolongs the duration of effective analgesia as compared to bupivacaine alone and delays the need for postoperative rescue analgesics without having any sedative effect, pruritus, or respiratory depression. The use of intrathecal midazolam also decreases the incidence of postoperative nausea vomiting (*PONV*). Moreover, intrathecal midazolam does not have any clinically significant effect on perioperative hemodynamics. A small diluted dose of preservative-free intrathecal midazolam *(<1mg/mL concentration and 1 to 2.5mg)* appears to have few systemic side effects and is free of short-term neurotoxicity.

4. Sedation in spinal anesthesia with intravenous midazolam

The use of spinal anesthesia is often limited by the unwillingness of patients to remain awake during surgery [69]. Spinal anesthesia provides anesthesia at the surgical site, yet unpleasant and uncomfortable patient experiences result from having to remain in the same position, prolonged duration of surgery or ambient noise in the operating room. To avoid spontaneous movements by an inadequately sedated patient that can interfere with the surgical procedure, intravenous sedative medications can be useful in patients who are positioned in specific postures that can be considered uncomfortable [70]. On the other hand, the goals of sedation during spinal anesthesia include rapid achievement of adequate sedation, its maintenance at a constant level during the surgical procedure and awakening the patient quickly at the end. This can be attained by continuous infusion of sedative drugs preceded by a bolus.

Conscious sedation is a minimally depressed level of consciousness that retains the patient's ability to maintain his or her airway independently and continuously, and to respond appropriately to physical stimulation and verbal command, produced by pharmacologic or non-pharmacologic methods, alone or in combination [71]. With conscious sedation only some of the centers in the medullary reticular formation and thalamus are depressed in a dose dependent manner [72]. Thus, this level of sedation provides the additional benefit of preservation of protective airway reflexes, especially in monitored anesthesia care. An ideal supplemental sedative should provide effective anxiolysis, an easily controllable level of sedation, predictable depth of amnesia, a rapid and clear headed recovery, minimal intraoperative side effects, no evidence of cumulation and minimal postoperative side effects. Numerous agents have been used as sedative adjuvants to spinal anesthesia, each with their own advantages and disadvantages.

The most widely used technique for administering sedation in regional anesthesia is the intermittent intravenous bolus dose technique. This technique has been shown to be associated with peaks and troughs in plasma concentration producing significant side effects and delayed recovery [73]. Continuous infusions have been proven to produce lesser side effects, faster recovery, easy controllability over the desired depth of sedation and, should the regional block prove to be ineffective, easy conversion to general anesthesia [74, 75].

Of the currently available benzodiazepines, midazolam has a fast onset and short recovery time, because of which it is one of the most widely used sedatives in spinal anesthesia. With a low context sensitive half time (*70 minutes for a four hour long infusion and up to 100 minutes for longer infusions*), it can be easily titrated to the needs of the patient, making its use well suited for ambulatory conscious sedation techniques [4, 76]. It produces good sedation and excellent amnesia but has no specific analgesic properties [77].

Benzodiazepines cause greater depression of upper airway muscle tone in the elderly, resulting in a higher incidence of airway obstruction [78, 79]. On the other hand, the synergistic effects between benzodiazepines and other drugs, especially opioids and propofol, facilitate better sedation and analgesia. However, the combination of these drugs also enhances their respiratory depression and may lead to airway obstruction or apnea [80]. Administration of oxygen to all the patients during sedation and immediate relief of airway obstruction prevented the occurrence of oxygen desaturation. A smaller volume bolus and a slow infusion rate avoided apnea.

Bolus administration of midazolam 0.05 mg/kg was reported to give enough amnesia and sedation without any adverse effects on hemodynamics and respiration [80]. With this method, patients did not respond to verbal command but recovered in 25 minutes [81] and opened their eyes spontaneously in 47 minutes [82]. As long as patients closed their eyes, amnesic effect was kept and when they opened their eyes, additional midazolam 1 mg (*approximately 18 mcg/kg*) was enough for patient's comfort [82]. However, bolus administration of sedative can not provide constant level of sedation. In contrast, continuous infusion can provide constant sedation level but usually prolongs onset time of sedation compared with the intermittent bolus technique [83]. Different studies showed that during spinal anesthesia, midazolam (*1-2 mg given and followed by 0.1-0.5 mg/kg/hr intravenously*) provides rapidly induced sedation and amnesia with stable hemodynamics and respiration. Oxygen must be administered at 3-6 L/min through a mask during the procedure. Intraoperative monitoring must include electrocardiography, pulse oxmetry, noninvasive sphygmomanometry, and capnography.

Midazolam is considered safe even at high doses and, at equipotent doses, it affects (*via GABA*) the central nervous system in a similar fashion [84]. GABA receptors are found in different parts of the brain. The sedative effects of the benzodiazepines are mediated by the brainstem GABA receptors that inhibit the ascending pathways that activate the brain cortex. The ataxia and memory impairment are mediated by GABA receptors in the cerebellar, hippocampal, and forebrain areas. While hypnosis or sedation is always achieved after appropriate individually based doses, anxiolysis is seldom transformed into anxiety, restlessness, rage or a myriad of uncontrolled behaviours (*midazolam paradox*)[84]. The relationship of the paradoxical reaction to alteration of the cholinergic homeostasis, serotonin levels, the role of genetics, and gamma-aminobutyric acid receptor configuration are suspect [85]. Such paradoxical reactions may harm the unconscious or semiconscious patient. Low dose of flumazenil (*0.2-0.3 mg, range 0.1-0.5 mg*) completely reverses midazolam-induced paradoxical reactions and they are more frequent in older patients [84, 85].

http://dx.doi.org/10.5772/58750

5. Conclusion

Spinal anesthesia has the advantage of being able to maintain spontaneous breathing as well as relaxing the necessary muscles for surgery. However, the time limit and patient's anxiety of spinal anesthesia are important disadvantages. On the other hand, the impediments to the effective use of spinal anesthesia are the predictable decreases in arterial blood pressure and heart rate through the accompanying sympathectomy with its attendant vasodilatation and blockade of cardio accelerator fibres. Another clinically important impediment to successful block is inadequate sedation. Adjunctive drugs are used to decrease anxiety, alleviate discomfort, improve hemodynamic stability and induce a feeling of calmness during spinal anesthesia.

When using sedative medication during spinal anesthesia, the anesthesiologist attempts to titrate the drug to optimize patient comfort while maintaining cardiorespiratory stability and intact protective reflexes. Morever, adequate sedation in spinal anesthesia relieves the anxiety of the patient, improves physiological and psychological stress, and increases the satisfaction of the surgeon, anesthetist and patient. Midazolam is most frequently used as the agent for sedation. It is often used intravenously in single doses of between 0.5 mg and 2.5 mg. Midazolam provides rapidly induced sedation and amnesia with stable hemodynamics and respiration during spinal anesthesia.

Moreover, midazolam has been shown to have antinociceptive effects when administered intrathecally, both in laboratory animals and in humans. Intrathecal injection up to 2 mg midazolam have been reported without adverse effects. The paucity of studies on intrathecal midazolam warrants caution in elderly patients, the obese, and those who are already on other sedatives. When intrathecal midazolam is used, all patients should be closely monitored intra and postoperatively. In brief, intrathecal preservative free midazolam appears safe and has clinically acceptable analgesic properties.

Author details

Beyazit Zencirci*

Marash Life Hospital – Department of Anesthesiology & Reanimation, Turkey

References

[1] Zencirci B. Postdural puncture headache and pregabalin. J Pain Res 2010;3:11-4.

[2] Ahmed F, Garg A, Chawla V, Khandelwal M. Transdermal nitroglycerine enhances postoperative analgesia of intrathecal neostigmine following abdominal hysterectomies. Indian J Anaesth 2010;54:24-8.

[3] Walser A, Benjamin LE, Flynn T, et al. Quinazolines and 1, 4-benzodiazepines. 84. Synthesis and reactions of imidazo[1, 5-a][1, 4]benzodiazepines. J Org Chem 1978;43:936-44.

[4] Reves JG, Fragen RJ, Vinik HR, Greenblatt DJ. Midazolam: pharmacology and uses. Anesthesiology 1985;62:310-24.

[5] Faull RL, Villiger JW. Benzodiazepine receptors in the human spinal cord: a detailed anatomical and pharmacological study. Neuroscience 1986;17:791-802.

[6] Goodchild CS, Serrao JM. Intrathecal midazolam in the rat: evidence for spinally-mediated analgesia. Br J Anaesth 1987;59:1563-70.

[7] Serrao JM, Marks RL, Morley SJ, Goodchild CS. Intrathecal midazolam for the treatment of chronic mechanical low back pain: a controlled comparison with epidural steroid in a pilot study. Pain 1992;48:5-12.

[8] Valentine JM, Lyons G, Bellamy MC. The effect of intrathecal midazolam on post-operative pain. Eur J Anaesthesiol 1996;13:589-93.

[9] Borg PA, Krijnen HJ. Long term intrathecal administration of midazolam and clonidine. Clin J Pain 1996;12:63-8.

[10] Goodchild CS, Guo Z, Musgreave A, Gent JP. Antinociception by intrathecal midazolam involves endogenous neurotransmitters acting at spinal cord delta opioid receptors. Br J Anaesth 1996;77:758-63.

[11] Olkkola KT, Ahonen J. Midazolam and other benzodiazepines. In: Schüttler J & Schwilden H. (eds) Handbook of Experimental Pharmacology (Volume-182, Modern Anesthetics). Berlin: Springer-Verlag; 2008. p.335-360.

[12] Eilers H. Intravenous anesthetics. In: Miller RD & Pardo MC. (eds.) Basics of Anesthesia 6th ed. Philadelphia: Elsevier Saunders; 2011. p99-114.

[13] Halliday NJ, Dundee JW, Collier PS, Loughran PG, Harper KW. Influence of plasma proteins on the onset of hypnotic action of intravenous midazolam. Anaesthesia 1985;40:763-66.

[14] Heizmann P, Eckert M, Ziegler WH. Pharmacokinetics and bioavailability of midazolam in man. Br J Clin Pharmacol 1983;16(Suppl 1):S43-S49.

[15] Greenblatt DJ, Abernethy DR, Locniskar A, et al. Effect of age, gender, and obesity in midazolam kinetics. Anesthesiology 1984;61:27-35.

[16] Harper KW, Collier PS, Dundee JW, et al. Age and nature of operation influence the pharmacokinetics of midazolam. Br J Anaesth 1985;57:866-71.

[17] Allonen H, Ziegler G, Klotz U. Midazolam kinetics. Clin Pharmacol Ther 1981;30:653-61.

[18] Greenblatt DJ, Shader RI, Franke K. Pharmacokinetics and bioavailability of intravenous, intramuscular, and oral lorazepam in humans. J Pharm Sci 1979;68:57-63.

[19] Dundee JW, Halliday NJ, Harper KW, Brogden RN. Midazolam. A review of its pharmacological properties and therapeutic use. Drugs 1984;28:519-54.

[20] Bailey L, Ward M, Musa MN. Clinical pharmacokinetics of benzodiazepines. J Clin Pharmacol 1994;34:804-11.

[21] Park GR, Manara AR, Dawling S. Extra-hepatic metabolism of midazolam. Br J Clin Pharmacol 1989;27:634-37.

[22] Pentikäinen PJ, Välisalmi L, Himberg JJ, Crevoicier C. Pharmacokinetics of midazolam following intravenous and oral administration in patients with chronic liver disease and in healthy subjects. J Clin Pharmacol 1989;29:272-77.

[23] Wandel C, Böcker R, Böhrer H, et al. Midazolam is metabolized by at least three different cytochrome P450 enzymes. Br J Anaesth 1994;73:658-61.

[24] Ziegler WH, Schalch E, Leishman B, Eckert M. Comparison of the effects of intravenously administered midazolam, triazolam and their hydroxyl metabolites. Br J Clin Pharmacol 1983;16(Suppl 1):S63-S69.

[25] Mandema JW, Tuk B, van Stevenick AL, et al. Pharmacokinetic-pharmacodynamic modelling of the central nervous system effects of midazolam and its main metabolite α-hydroxymidazolam in healthy volunteers. Clin Pharmacol Ther 1992;51:715-28.

[26] Bauer TM, Ritz R, Haberthür C, et al. Prolonged sedation due to accumulation of conjugated metabolites of midazolam. Lancet 1995;346(8968):145-47.

[27] Greenblatt DJ, Shader RI, Abernethy DR. Drug therapy. Current status of benzodiazepines, N Engl J Med 1983;309:354-58.

[28] Arendt RM, Greenblatt DJ, deJong RH, et al. In vitro correlates of benzodiazepine cerebrospinal fluid uptake, pharmacodynamic action and peripheral distribution. J Pharmacol Exp Ther 1983;227:98-106.

[29] Mendelson WB. Neuropharmacology of sleep induction by benzodiazepines. Crit Rev Neurobiol 1992;6:221-32.

[30] Strange PG. D1/D2 dopamine receptor interaction at the biochemical level. Trends Pharmacol Sci 1991;12:48-9.

[31] Möhler H, Fritschy JM, Rudolph U. A new benzodiazepine pharmacology. J Pharmacol Exp Ther 2002;300:2-8.

[32] Tan PH, Chia YY, Lo Y, et al. Intrathecal bupivacaine with morphine or neostigmine for postoperative analgesia after total knee replacement. Can J Anaesth 2001;48:551-56.

[33] Kathirvel S, Sadhasivam S, Saxena A, Kannan TR, Ganjoo P. Effects of intrathecal ketamine added to bupivacaine for spinal anaesthesia. Anaesthesia 2000;55:899-904.

[34] Dobrydnjov I, Axelsson K, Samarütel J, Holmström B. Postoperative pain relief following intrathecal bupivacaine combined with intrathecal or oral clonidine. Acta Anaesthesiol Scand 2002;46:806-14.

[35] Prakash S, Joshi N, Gogia AR, Prakash S, Singh R. Analgesic efficacy of two doses of intrathecal midazolam with bupivacaine in patients undergoing cesarean delivery. Reg Anesth Pain Med 2006;31:221-26.

[36] Goodchild CS, Noble J. The effect of intrathecal midazolam on sympathetic nervous system reflexes in man-a pilot study. Br J Clin Pharmacol 1987;23:279-85.

[37] Yegin A, Sanli S, Dosemeci L, et al. The analgesic and sedative effects of intrathecal midazolam in perianal surgery. Eur J Anaesthesiol 2004;21:658-62.

[38] Tony LY, Jeffrey WA. The use of intrathecal midazolam in humans: a case study of process. Anesth Analg 2004;98:1536-45.

[39] Buchheit T, Rauck R. Subarachnoid techniques for cancer pain therapy: When, why, and how? Curr Rev Pain 1999;3:198-205.

[40] Bohlhalter S, Weinmann O, Mohler H, Fritschy JM. Laminar compartmentalization of GABAA-receptor subtypes in the spinal cord: an immunohistochemical study. J Neurosci 1996;16:283-97.

[41] Niv D, Whitwam JG, Loh L. Depression of nociceptive sympathetic reflexes by the intrathecal administration of midazolam. Br J Anaesth 1983;55:541-47.

[42] Edwards M, Serrao JM, Gent JP, Goodchild CS. On the mechanism by which midazolam causes spinally mediated analgesia. Anesthesiology 1990;73:273-77.

[43] Malinovsky JM, Cozian A, Lepage JY, et al. Ketamine and midazolam neurotoxicity in the rabbit. Anesthesiology 1991;75:91-7.

[44] Erdine S, Yücel A, Ozyalçin S, et al. Neurotoxicity of midazolam in the rabbit. Pain 1999;80:419-23.

[45] Schoeffler P, Auroy P, Bazin JE, Taxi J, Woda A. Subarachnoid midazolam: histologic study in rats and report of its effect on chronic pain in humans. Reg Anesth 1991;16:329-32.

[46] Aguilar JL, Espachs P, Roca G, et al. Difficult management of pain following sacrococcygeal chordoma: 13 months of subarachnoid infusion. Pain 1994;59:317-20.

[47] Svensson BA, Welin M, Gordh T Jr, Westman J. Chronic subarachnoid midazolam (Dormicum) in the rat. Morphologic evidence of spinal cord neurotoxicity. Reg Anesth 1995;20:426-34.

[48] Bozkurt P, Tunali Y, Kaya G, Okar I. Histological changes following epidural injection of midazolam in the neonatal rabbit. Paediatr Anaesth 1997;7:385-89.

[49] Bahar M, Cohen ML, Grinshpon Y, Chanimov M. Spinal anaesthesia with midazolam in the rat. Can J Anaesth 1997;44:208-15.

[50] Nishiyama T, Matsukawa T, Hanaoka K. Acute phase histopathological study of spinally administered midazolam in cats. Anesth Analg 1999;89:717-20.

[51] Nishiyama T, Matsukawa T, Hanaoka K. Continuous epidural administration of midazolam and bupivacaine forpostoperative analgesia. Acta Anaesthesiol Scand 1999;43:568-72.

[52] Nishiyama T, Sugai N, Hanaoka K. In vitro changes in the transparency and pH of cerebrospinal fluid caused by adding midazolam. Eur J Anaesthesiol 1998;15:27-31.

[53] Güleç S, Büyükkidan B, Oral N, Ozcan N, Tanriverdi B. Comparison of caudal bupivacaine, bupivacaine-morphine and bupivacaine-midazolam mixtures for post-operative analgesia in children. Eur J Anaesthesiol 1998;15:161-65.

[54] Batra YK, Jain K, Chari P, et al. Addition of intrathecal midazolam to bupivacaine produces better post-operative analgesia without prolonging recovery. Int J Clin Pharmacol Ther 1999;37:519-23.

[55] Kim MH, Lee YM. Intrathecal midazolam increases the analgesic effects of spinal blockade with bupivacaine in patients undergoing haemorrhoidectomy. Br J Anaesth 2001;86:77-9.

[56] Sen A, Rudra A, Sarkar SK, Biswas B. Intrathecal midazolam for postoperative pain relief in caesarean section delivery. J Indian Med Assoc 2001;99:683-86.

[57] Mahajan R, Batra YK, Grover VK, Kajal J. A comparative study of caudal bupivacaine and midazolam-bupivacaine mixture for post-operative analgesia in children undergoing genitourinary surgery. Int J Clin Pharmacol Ther 2001;39:116-20.

[58] Shah FR, Halbe AR, Panchal ID, Goodchild CS. Improvement in postoperative pain relief by the addition of midazolam to an intrathecal injection of buprenorphine and bupivacaine. Eur J Anaesthesiol 2003;20:904-10.

[59] Bharti N, Madan R, Mohanty PR, Kaul HL. Intrathecal midazolam added to bupivacaine improves the duration and quality of spinal anaesthesia. Acta Anaesthesiol Scand 2003;47:1101-05.

[60] Tucker AP, Lai C, Nadeson R, Goodchild CS. Intrathecal midazolam I: a cohort study investigating safety. Anesth Analg 2004;98:1512-20.

[61] Tucker AP, Mezzatesta J, Nadeson R, Goodchild CS. Intrathecal midazolam II: combination with intrathecal fentanyl for labor pain. Anesth Analg 2004;98:1521-27.

[62] Prochazka J. 775 intrathecal midazolam as an analgesic—10 years experience. Eur J Pain 2006;10(Suppl 1):S202.

[63] Gupta A, Prakash S, Deshpande S, Kale KS. The effect of intrathecal midazolam 2.5 mg with hyperbaric bupivacaine on postoperative pain relief in patients undergoing orthopedic surgery. The Internet Journal of Anesthesiology 2007;14. http://ispub.com/IJA/14/2/3671 (accesed 11 August 2013).

[64] Ho KM, Ismail H. Use of intrathecal midazolam to improve perioperative analgesia: a meta-analysis. Anesth Intensive Care 2008;36:365-73.

[65] Yun MJ, Kim YH, Kim JH, et al. Intrathecal midazolam added to bupivacaine prolongs the duration of spinal blockade to T10 dermatome in orthopedic patients. Korean J Anesthesiol 2007;53:S22-S28.

[66] Jaiswal S, Ranjan P, Tewari N, Agarwal NR, Mathur S. Comparative study of epidural midazolam and butorphanol as adjuvant with bupivacaine for labor analgesia: A double blind study. The Internet Journal of Anesthesiology 2007;14. http://ispub.com/IJA/14/1/10602 (accesed 11 August 2013).

[67] Agrawal N, Usmani A, Sehgal R, Kumar R, Bhadoria P. Effect of intrathecal midazolam bupivacaine combination on postoperative analgesia. Indian J Anaesth 2005;49:37-9.

[68] Shadangi BK, Garg R, Pandey R, Das T. Effects of intrathecal midazolam in spinal anaesthesia: a prospective randomised case control study. Singapore Med J 2011;52:432-35.

[69] Wu CL, Naqibuddin M, Fleisher LA. Measurement of patient satisfaction as an outcome of regional anesthesia and analgesia: a systematic review. Reg Anesth Pain Med 2001;26:196-208.

[70] De Andrés J, Valía JC, Gil A, Bolinches R. Predictors of patient satisfaction with regional anesthesia. Reg Anesth 1995;20:498-505.

[71] Practice guidelines for sedation and analgesia by non-anesthesiologists. American Society of Anesthesiologists Task Force on Sedation and Analgesia by Non-Anesthesiologists. Anesthesiology 2002;96:1004-17.

[72] Drummond JC. Monitoring depth of anesthesia: with emphasis on the application of the bispectral index and the middle latency auditory evoked response to the prevention of recall. Anesthesiology 2000;93:876-82.

[73] Höhener D, Blumenthal S, Borgeat A. Sedation and regional anaesthesia in the adult patient. Br J Anaesth 2008;100:8-16.

[74] Smith I, Monk TG, White PF, Ding Y. Propofol infusion during regional anesthesia: sedative, amnestic, and anxiolytic properties. Anesth Analg 1994;79:313-19.

[75] Casati A, Fanelli G, Casaletti E, et al. Clinical assessment of target-controlled infusion of propofol during monitored anesthesia care. Can J Anaesth 1999;46:235-39.

[76] Stoelting RK, Hillier SC. Benzodiazepines. In: Stoelting RK & Hillier SC. (eds.). Pharmacology and Physiology in Anesthetic Practice 4th ed, Philadelphia: Lippincott Williams & Wilkins, 2006. p140-54.

[77] de Andrés J, Bolinches R. Comparative study of propofol and midazolam for sedation in regional anesthesia. Rev Esp Anestesiol Reanim 1993;40:354-59.

[78] Leiter JC, Knuth SL, Krol RC, Bartlett D Jr. The effect of diazepam on genioglossal muscle activity in normal human subjects. Am Rev Respir Dis 1985;132:216-19.

[79] Montravers P, Dureuil B, Desmonts JM. Effects of i.v. midazolam on upper airway resistance. Br J Anaesth 1992;68:27-31.

[80] Bailey PL, Pace NL, Ashburn MA, et al. Frequent hypoxemia and apnea after sedation with midazolam and fentanyl. Anesthesiology 1990;73:826-30.

[81] Nishiyama T, Hirasaki A, Odaka Y, Iwasaki T, Seto K. Midazolam sedation during spinal anesthesia: Optimal dosage. J Jpn Soc Clin Anesth 1994;14:257-62.

[82] Nishiyama T, Hanaoka K. The necessity and the efficacy of the second administration of midazolam for sedation during spinal anesthesia. Masui 2000;49:245-49.

[83] White PF. Use of continuous infusion versus intermittent bolus administration of fentanyl or ketamine during outpatient anesthesia. Anesthesiology 1983;59:294-300.

[84] Weinbroum AA, Szold O, Ogorek D, Flaishon R. The midazolam-induced paradox phenomenon is reversible by flumazenil. Epidemiology, patient characteristics and review of the literature. Eur J Anaesthesiol 2001;18:789-97.

[85] Robin C, Trieger N. Paradoxical reactions to benzodiazepines in intravenous sedation: a report of 2 cases and review of the literature. Anesth Prog 2002;49:128-32.

Chapter 7

Complications in Spinal Anaesthesia

Alparslan Apan and Özgün Cuvaş Apan

Additional information is available at the end of the chapter

http://dx.doi.org/10.5772/58817

1. Introduction

Spinal anaesthesia is one of the most popular and widely used anaesthetic procedures. It is a simple, cost effective and efficient technique that provides complete sensory and motor block, as well as postoperative analgaesia with a high success rate. Several advantages of spinal anaesthesia include a decreased incidence of deep vein thrombosis, reduced intraoperative blood loss, as well as the prevention of pulmonary aspiration in case of emergency, especially in patients with potential airway problems and known respiratory diseases.

Due to the invasive nature of spinal anaesthesia, there are several types of complications that may occur with different incidence. At least some of these problems appear to be inevitable and as such, it is not possible to eliminate them all. Fortunately, more severe neurological complications such as death, neuropathy, arachnoiditis and permanent neurologic injury are seldom observed. In a national survey performed in the UK, the incidence of permanent neurologic injury and death ranged from 0. 7 to 1. 8 in 100, 000 patients [1]. On the other hand, proper patient selection, meticulous attention to detail, well-known patient related changes and in the case of difficult circumstances, using image techniques [x rays, fluoroscopy and ultrasound] as a guide may help to prevent or decrease complications.

Increasing co-morbidities, concomitant medication, surgery for advanced malignancy, patients with compromised immune systems, as well as instances of infection poses a real challenge to the use of spinal anaesthesia. Patients with degenerative vertebral anomalies or who have undergone previous spinal surgeries are also difficult cases; these require further evaluation and an increase in efforts for properly performing intrathecal anaesthesia and analgaesia in contexts where it may lead to undesirable consequences.

2. Hypotension

Hypotension is an inevitable complication of spinal anaesthesia that occurs when the sympathetic chain becomes blocked, especially when higher dermatome levels are needed. A drop in blood pressure may initiate nausea and vomiting, indicating ischaemia on the spinal cord, which in turn induces an undesired condition for the patient and operating staff. Blood pressure changes between the left lateral to supine position has been determined as an indicator for predicting a perioperative decrease in obstetric patients undergoing caesarean delivery under spinal anaesthesia [2].

In a non-obstetric study population, changing patients to the Trendelenburg position for 10 minutes immediately following a spinal block has been demonstrated as efficient, as has loading with a lactated ringer or 6% hydroxyl ethyl starch solution by means of maintaining cardiac output. Co-hydration is more efficient than pre-hydration and colloid loading is better for maintaining cardiac output and blood pressure [3]. In their report, Shin et al. [4] investigated the influence of crystalloid and colloid loading on cerebrospinal fluid movements in volunteers, as well as the spread of local anaesthetics in patients. Although crystalloid pre-treatment delayed the cranial spread of the block, it induced cerebrospinal fluid production, which may be valuable in the case of post-dural-puncture headache [PDPH].

In case of pregnancy, a decrease in blood pressure at the critical level may affect both mother and baby, and result in more serious outcomes over a longer period. Increased venodilatation under the influence of progesterone or prostaglandins may also contribute to changes in blood pressure. The presence of hypertension, advanced age, increased body mass index, higher birth weight and higher block are considered as risk factors in hypotension performed with spinal anaesthesia. Fluid loading, lateral tilt or wedge performed under the right buttock to prevent aortocaval compression, or vasopressor therapy, constitutes preventive measurements to treat hypotension in obstetric patients. The influence of aortocaval pressure or other determinants remain controversial in terms of how they contribute to haemodynamics during spinal anaesthesia. In order to attenuate the effect of hypotension, the influence of positioning the patient on a lateral decubitus position for a brief period was investigated. The hypotension episode showed a slight delay, but the incidence of hypotension or drug use was the same as observed in patients lying supine] [5]. In an editorial, Sharwood-Smith and Drummond [6] criticized the role of vena caval compression in light of the presence of persistent vasoconstriction, such as observed in patients with pre-eclampsia, which is known to be volume depleted or hypovolemic; hypotension, however, was observed to a lesser extent. These observations justify vasopressor therapy and indicate that sympathetic block affecting arterial vasculature might be a major concern related to arterial pressure drop [6].

Time, duration and the selection of vasoactive drugs are controversial issues where obstetric patients are concerned. Ephedrine may stimulate beta adrenergic receptors by crossing the umbilical cord and increasing foetal acidosis; therefore, phenylephrine has become the vasopressor of choice [7]. Variable infusion has been demonstrated as being superior to the fixed infusion and 25-50 $\mu g\ min^{-1}$ was demonstrated to be sufficient or maintaining hemodynamic status. Non-invasive cardiac output monitoring might be indicated for a patient with severe cardiac disease [8]. On the other hand, a phenylephrine infusion may induce bradycardia, presumed (or) indicated by the baroreflex receptor mediated mechanism [9].

3. Hypothermia

A decrease in body temperature is commonly encountered after neuraxial anaesthesia. Subarachnoid local anaesthetic administration blocks all afferents of skin temperature that patients are unable to release the decrease in core temperature. Vasodilation due to sympathetic blockade increases skin blood flow, which allows for lowering the body's core temperature in a reliable manner. In preparing the skin for surgery with antiseptic solutions, especially when performed on a large area, evaporation from surgical field and irrigation solutions, or fluid infusion at a higher rate, may also contribute to hypothermia during surgery. [Fig 1] A decrease in core temperature may initiate shivering, especially during the postoperative period, which increases oxygen consumption. Hypothermia is known to induce hyper coagulation and infections. Special care should be exerted to decrease this physiologic stress, especially in paediatric, obstetric and patients in advanced age, since it may lead to serious consequences, including low perfusion to the vital organs, coronary ischaemia and infection [10].

It is crucial to warm the patient with blankets, surgical thermal mattresses, forced air heathers, by using pre-warmed irrigation, intravenous solutions and blood products in order to decrease the severity of this complication.

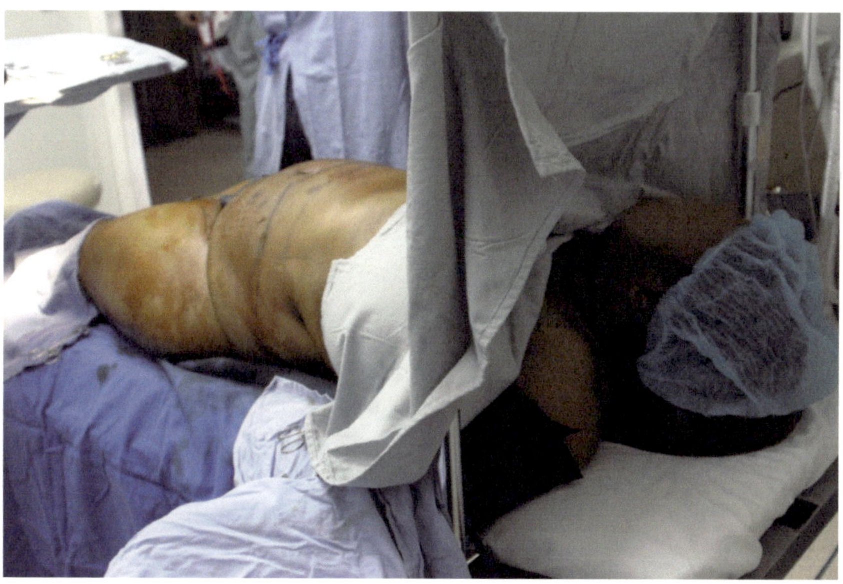

Figure 1. Large areas of skin prepped with a Povidone-iodine solution and uncovered during surgery favour hypothermia and its complications [Source: www. anestesia-dolor. org].

4. Post-dural-puncture headache

PDPH is a troublesome complication, mostly observed in middle-aged women and the obstetric population. Lower body mass index, previous PDPH and the presence of chronic headaches are other risk factors. Headache rarely occurs in the paediatric population, especially in neonates, but some physicians believe that this may be due to the inability to communicate pain in early childhood. PDPH also decreases with age, which may be related to changes in the composition of cerebral content, which increase on cerebrospinal fluid [CSF] that may compensate and prevents its occurrence.

PDPH requires differentiation from other causes of headache [11]. It typically occurs in the fronto-occipital region with nuchal rigidity and initiates when moving from the supine position to sitting or standing up. It may vary from mild to severe and the type of pain may be dull, throbbing or burning. Vertigo, nausea and vomiting might be observed due to PDPH in some patients. Headache typically appears on the second day following the dural puncture and can range from lasting one to four days, but may be observed as early as 20 min after the dural puncture [12]. The leaking of CSF across the dural hole may initiate PDPH. This is explained by the following mechanisms: a decrease in intracranial pressure causes the traction of pain sensitive cranial structures, the depletion of CSF volume may induce compensatory cerebral vasodilatation [the Monroe-Kelly doctrine] and the activation of adenosine receptors may cause cerebral vasodilatation [13].

The incidence of PDPH has been reported at a level of 2.5% when using a 25 G pencil point needle in obstetric patients [14]; in the non-obstetric population, the incidence of PDPH is as low as 0.37% when using fine spinal needles [15]. Cutting edge needles are not recommended for spinal anaesthesia, due to the increased incidence of PDPH, even when using fine needles in patients undergoing anorectal surgery [16].

Accidental dural entry is a more distressing event that occurs while advancing the Tuohy needle or epidural catheter, resulting in PDPH at a level of about 75%. The epidural catheter is presumed to introduce from weak points of dura which may occurs with Tuohy needle Incidence of this occurring has been reported as 0.5% in an obstetrical referral centre [17]. It is not possible to recognize or observe clear CSF in needles or catheters in all patients. Therefore, as a treatment tool, re-inserting the epidural catheter in a different lumbar interspace, or leaving the catheter in the perforated dura mater with the intent to decrease PDPH does not succeed in all patients.

Patient position when performing spinal anaesthesia, the experience of the physician and using finer needles do not appear to influence the occurrence of PDPH [17]. Pneumocephalus with subsequent PDPH is a rare but well-described complication of unintentional dural puncture. It has late clinical onset manifestations and can induce a long-lasting headache as a result of accidental dural entry when epidural anaesthesia is performed by means of the loss of resistance technique, using air [18].

The treatment algorithm depends on the severity of PDPH. Conservative treatment consists of bed rest and oral or intravenous fluid replacement. Pharmacological therapy includes analgaesics, vasoconstrictors or drugs that increase CSF production. Paracetamol or non-steroidal anti-inflammatory drugs are used as first step treatment. Vasoconstrictors, such as caffeine and Sumatripan, have been used but with limited benefits. Caffeine should be prescribed with caution due to the patient having a lowered convulsion threshold and long term administration is not advised. Gabapentin has also been used successfully for the treatment of PDPH. Drug therapy may provide relief, but do not completely resolve the symptoms. Epidural morphine has also been demonstrated as beneficial but may leak from the dural hole into the intrathecal space and has well-known side effects such as pruritus, nausea and vomiting [19].

Although controversies surrounding it remain, the epidural blood patch [EBP] remains the gold standard for treating PDPH. A sterile sample of 15-20 mL autologous blood is drawn from the patient and immediately injected at the same or a lower level inside the epidural space, until backache or dullness can be felt. It is generally performed after waiting 24 hours following the epidural block. If PDPH persists, a second EBP a week later may be necessary. A third EBP is seldom needed. In a series of cases, the volume of blood needed was reduced while performing EBP under fluoroscopy guidance [20].

The witnessed accidental dural entry has different treatment options. Advancing an epidural catheter to the subarachnoid space, injecting 10 mL of saline initially and leaving the catheter in place for 24 hours are helpful for decreasing the incidence of PDPH. A catheter is believed to induce inflammatory reaction to the dural hole and closure may occur during withdrawal of catheter. At the very least, the presence of the epidural catheter may impede CSF leakage. Epidural catheter placement in a different interspace has also shown potential benefits. Epidural saline or a dextran infusion for creating a fluid column has limited therapeutic efficacy, possibly due to the easy reabsorption from dural veins [21]. Fibrin glue was also used, especially in patients who refuted the therapy or any other contraindications such as coexisting systemic infection [22]. Surgical treatment is the final step; this only occurs if chronic leakage persists [23].

Cranial hypotension and long-lasting CSF loss may distract cerebral bridging veins that can easily rupture and lead to acute or chronic subdural or subarachnoid haematoma occurring. Caution should be applied when spinal anaesthesia is implemented in a patient who has experienced recent cranial trauma, the likes of which may either facilitate or confuse the outcome. Neurological investigation should be performed when the headache lasts more than a few days and is resistant to the conservative treatment [2]. Spinal haematoma is a rare event that may relate to the direct needle trauma [25].

Chronic leakage and cranial hypotension may influence cranial nerves and nerve palsies may rarely occur due to compression or altered blood supply. It mostly affects the VI cranial nerve; the reason for this might be attributed to its longer course (or path) in cranium [26]. Treatment modalities against CSF leakage and specific therapy for nerve palsy, including corticosteroids, have been demonstrated as being beneficial [27]. Altered mental status and speech or stupor may be observed with intracranial hypotension, headache, nausea and vomiting, and determined as posterior reversible encephalopathy syndrome presenting as oedema in the posterior cerebral portions with MRI. This syndrome is largely related to the systemic illness that was first described in an obstetric patient following spinal anaesthesia. The late onset and course of the syndrome implicates compression of posterior portion of the brain vault due to chronic loss of CSF [28]. Reversible cerebral vasoconstrictor syndrome is another entity that has similar clinical features such as headache but lacks imaging findings [29].

Hearing loss is another complication related to loss of CSF during spinal anaesthesia. Hearing disability especially affects low frequencies on audiometry and commonly occurs at the second post spinal block. Studies have shown that aims to decrease incidences of leaking CSF using fine and pencil-point-tipped spinal needles can decrease this complication [30]. Type intravenous fluid loading either using crystalloid or colloid do not seems to largely influence or prevents the presence of auditory malfunctions [31].

5. Transient neurologic symptoms

Radicular symptoms, including pain, a burning sensation on the buttocks, dysaesthesia and paraesthesia may be observed following spinal anaesthesia. These symptoms generally subside within two days. But these clinical features are alarming for possible serious consequences. There is no representation of these symptoms on radiographs, CT or MRI. Ambulatory surgery, lithotomy position, the type of local anaesthetic used, as well as the concentration of dextrose and osmolarity has being mentioned as contributing factors for transient neurologic symptoms. The use of spinal lidocaine is one factor that may increase the incidence of transient neurologic symptoms, especially when some factors are combined. An increase in local anaesthetic concentration by pooling and maldistribution may also increase the incidence of this complication [32]. In a review by Zaric et al. [33], the authors indicated that the relative risk was about seven-to eight-fold lower with other local anaesthetics such as bupivacaine, mepivacaine, and prilocaine.

6. Urinary retention

Bladder distension during the postoperative period produces discomfort to patients and unless relieved, leads to more severe complications, including permanent injury to the detrusor muscle. Spinal anaesthesia influences urination by blocking all afferent nerve fibres, rendering the patient unable to feel bladder distension or urinary urgency. Bladder catheterization is not innocuous; it carries the risk of urethral trauma and more severe complications, including infection and haematologic spread that may reach the surgical site [34]. Urodynamic studies indicate that the function of the detrusor muscle returns to normal after about 100 min longer than the sensorial level regression from the S2 to S3 level [35]. It has been demonstrated that spontaneous urination may be influenced by an intrathecal local anaesthetic; long-acting agents require a longer time to recover from urinary function [36].

Several surgical risk factors may increase the incidence of urinary retention, such as anorectal surgery, inguinal hernia, orthopaedic [especially hip] surgery, abdominal surgery, instrumental delivery, prolongation of labour and gynaecologic surgery [37]. Patient characteristics showed that being predisposed to urinary retention included the male gender, 50 years and older and the presence of urination problems [38]. Besides neuraxial anaesthesia, some of the anaesthesia-related or intraoperative factors are prolongation of anaesthesia or surgery, increased intraoperative fluid volume [>750 mL], a required atropine, decreased body temperature and opioid-based anaesthesia, which may increase urinary retention [38, 39]. Spinal anaesthesia may also contribute to this complication by increasing or contributing to the requirements of at least several factors mentioned above.

Commonly used additives such as opioids or epinephrine may also increase the time leading up to urinating. In a meta-analysis, hydrophilic opioids were more prone to contribute to urinary retention than lipophilic compounds, which are especially important for outpatient surgery [40]. The gap between general anaesthesia and neuraxial blocks are decreased when systemic opioids are predominantly used for pain control [38]. The duration of spinal anaesthesia performed with hyperbaric local anaesthetics is shorter than more plain solutions, which may also be preferred [41]. Interestingly, when compared to the same intrathecal dose, more dilute solutions of local anaesthetics regressed earlier and regained bladder function faster [42]. Short-acting local anaesthetics, the administration of which should be given in as low a dose as possible, a plain or hyperbaric solution with no additives and avoiding an unnecessary increase of sensorial levels may decrease this complication in susceptible individuals within the outpatient setting. Indeed, a meticulous review indicates that there is no risk involved in single shot spinal anaesthesia when such precautions are taken [43]. Bladder volume is also an important issue during admission to the intensive care unit. Single bladder catheterization may be necessary during the peri-operative period or immediately following surgery. Ultrasound may precisely determine the bladder volume in adults and can be an important part of routine use in post-anaesthesia care units [44]. A multimodal approach for postoperative pain regarding the decrease of systemic opioids might be beneficial to avoid unnecessary hospital re-admissions. Non opioids, non-steroid anti-inflammatory drugs and other regional techniques such as wound infiltration and peripheral nerve blocks have also been demonstrated to decrease urinary retention [43].

7. Haematologic complications

Spinal haematoma following spinal anaesthesia is a severe complication that requires early surgical intervention to prevent permanent neurological damage. Classically, the incidence of this condition has been accepted as 1 in 220, 000 patients undergoing spinal anaesthesia, but the actual incidence remains unknown and is presumed to be on the increase. Advanced age, female gender, patients receiving drugs that influence coagulation, difficulty in performing block and placement of the indwelling epidural catheter are mentioned as risk factors [45]. A study investigating neurologic complications after neuraxial block, performed in Sweden over a period of ten years, indicates an increased incidence in female patients undergoing hip fracture surgery – 1 in 22, 000 compared to 1 in 480, 000 when all patients were included [46]. Haematoma was more frequently encountered with epidural anaesthesia or catheter placement, because of the increased vascularity of the epidural space. The presence of haematoma is frequently suspected in the case of an unexpected increase in the duration of motor block or delay on recovery. Neurosurgery within eight hours after the epidural haematoma is mandatory to regain motor functions without neurologic harm. Should neurologic harm be suspected, imaging studies, including computed tomography or preferably MRI, should be implemented as early as possible. Unfortunately, neurologic outcomes have been poor for the majority of patients, even when surgery was performed within eight hours. Spinal catheters should be considered as epidural catheters, for which placement or removal requires strict adherence to withdrawal guidelines to avoid having an effect on anticoagulation therapy.

Many drugs interfere with blood clotting, thereby requiring adherence to recommendations for the removal of neuraxial catheters. A number of regional anaesthesia societies have published their own recommendations [47, 48, 49]. Recent evidence indicates spinal anaesthesia to be safe, provided the half-life of the drug or residual effects are monitored. Non-steroidal anti-inflammatory drugs are considered safe, but concomitant drug use can increase the risk of haematoma. Therefore, patients receiving more than one drug affecting coagulation should be carefully evaluated. Additionally, some herbal drugs only or in combination with anticoagulants can increase the risk of spinal haematoma [45].

Central neuraxial blocks in patients with pre-existing haematologic disorders or disease affecting coagulation do not appear to be a significant problem. In their review, Choi and Brull [50] investigated the outcome of neuroaxial anaesthesia in patients with common bleeding disorders. A total of 78 spinal anaesthetics, 53 diagnostic lumbar punctures and two combined spinal and epidural anaesthetics were performed. No bleeding complications were observed, except in one infant, who was an unknown haemophilia A, developed spinal haematoma and needed surgical decompression. Spinal anaesthesia appears to be safe in patients with known bleeding disorders, provided that the status of coagulation is monitored. Although there is no consensus concerning a safe platelet count, 50, 000 to 80, 000 mm^3 is generally considered a critical number for spinal or epidural anaesthesia. Individual patient assessment should be conducted in patients with lower platelet counts [51]. For more details, the reader is referred to the chapter on spinal haematoma included in this book.

8. Infectious complications

Although bacterial meningitis following neuraxial anaesthesia is an uncommon complication, in cases where it does occur it may result in severe harm, including permanent neurologic disability and death. The presence of a fever and neurologic disturbance may provide a differentiation from PDPH. Epidural abscess is generally caused by skin flora; the bacteria most frequently involved is *S. aureus*. It is therefore prudent to initiate treatment with synthetic penicillin, even in the absence of a positive culture. Other less common causes of infection are aerobic and anaerobic streptococci, and anaerobic gram-negative bacilli. The incidence of meningitis varies between 1 in 50, 000 and mostly occurs as a result of airborne pathogens. The exact mechanism for how the microorganism reaches the spinal cord remains controversial. It may occur during preparation or performing the block, with a droplet from medical personal is the predominant source. Infection is more likely to occur in streptococci in most of the cases, emphasizing the need for strict adherence to precautions while performing spinal anaesthesia [52].

A case report and review from the literature indicates 179 cases of bacterial meningitis related to the central neuraxial puncture for any indication covering the period 1952 to 2005, in which 54% was related to spinal anaesthesia and 5% was observed for the combined spinal and epidural technique, which included 15 obstetric patients. Technical difficulties during placement of the needle or repeated attempts to spinal anaesthesia appear to be contributing factors [53].

Spinal anaesthesia in patients with coexisting infection is a controversial issue. In their study, Gritsenko et al. [54] retrospectively reviewed patients who had undergone removal of an infected prosthesis due to hip or knee arthroplasty performed under neuraxial anaesthesia to look for possible associations between perioperative infection and postoperative neuraxial complications regarding meningitis or epidural abscess. Although higher incidence of positive joint culture or pus was found during these procedures, none of the patients included in the 474 cases demonstrated infectious complications during the postoperative period. A study performed by Bader et al. [55] investigated 319 obstetric patients with chorioamnionitis, eight of whom had bacteraemia, but none developed neuraxial infection following neuraxial anaesthesia. A similar study of 517 patients with the same pathology, including 13 cases of systemic infection, demonstrated no meningitis or epidural abscess [56]. These results indicate that the possibility of haematologic spread through the spinal cord from the remote site as an infectious source is less likely to occur; regardless, clinicians are advised to perform the block under empirical antibacterial therapy.

Spinal anaesthesia in a patient with immunodeficiency is another instance where the presence of infection has been observed to lead to positive CSF culture and infection [57]. Therefore, performing spinal anaesthesia in such patients requires strict attention and may be attempted in combination with antibiotic treatment.

On the other hand, in a large prospective study including obstetric patients, general anaesthesia was associated with a higher incidence of surgical site infection and post-operative hospital stay compared to the use of spinal or epidural blocks [58].

9. Neurologic complications

A review by Brull et al. [59], which included a large series of neurologic complications, reported that the incidence of permanent neurological injury following spinal anaesthesia varied between 0 to 4. 2per 10 000 patients. In a French survey, permanent neurological injury other than that caused by haemorrhage was more common and included injury to the conus medullaris, and the estimated risk was calculated as 1:78 660 spinal anaesthesia patients; incidence was nearly half the amount in obstetric patients compared to the non-obstetric population. Pre-existing spinal pathology or disease increases the incidence of postoperative neurologic complications following neuraxial blockade. Repeated attempts or improper positioning of patients may facilitate neurologic injury [60]. Lumbar canal stenosis is another contributing factor for adverse neurologic outcome [61]. The presence of scoliosis with or without prior surgery constitutes difficulties for performing neuraxial anaesthesia. When compared to spinal blocks, the success rate was lower with epidural anaesthesia, due to technical difficulties and improper distribution of local anaesthetics [62]. Although the precise mechanism was not determined, hydrostatic pressure performed during an epidural block was indicated as a possible source of injury. On the other hand, direct needle trauma appears to be one of the preventable reasons for neurological complications. It is best to withdraw the needle in the case of paraesthesia, which is highly associated with postoperative radiculopathy and repeating local anaesthetic injection should be avoided in order to prevent toxic concentrations in the spinal cord [63].

Reynolds [64] reported a series of cases of conus medullaris injury that including one non-obstetric and six obstetric female patients, resulting in long-lasting neurologic damage. Spinal anaesthesia was performed in three of the patients, while combined spinal and epidural anaesthesia was accomplished in the rest of the other patients. Only one patient suffered pain during needle placement. The possible reasons for this were indicated as misplacement of the needle at the lower end of the spinal cord, misidentification ofTuffier's line or that the arachnoid membrane may have been attached to the conus like a web. Author concluded that Tuffier's line was an unreliable method for identifying the correct intervertebral level [64]. Possibly, the addition of cutaneous and subcutaneous tissue over the crista iliaca in obese patients, or in the case of pregnancy, may erroneously lead to performing a higher intervertebral space for needle placement. Indeed, Broadbent et al. [65] demonstrated that an anaesthesiologist incorrectly identified the correct intervertebral space by palpation. Assuming the correct intervertebral space was correct in only 30% of patients using palpation and in 71% using ultrasound [66]. In a MRI study of 690 patients, Kim et al. [67] indicated that caution should be exercised when selecting the appropriate intervertebral space, especially in obese and elderly patients. The level of conus medullaris might be lower than expected in female patients with thoracic vertebral compression fractures [68]. These points have also been highlighted along with determining lateral needle deviation or placement as a source of possible reasons for neurological injury in a study group by the American Society of Regional Anesthesia [ASRA]; clinicians are advised to especially be aware of challenging surface anatomical changes [69]. Ultrasound imaging can also be used to guide proper accomplishment of neuraxial anaesthesia. Although promising results have been published on facilitating neuroaxial anaesthesia in difficult cases by means of decreasing the time and number of attempts [70], to date, it is not yet possible to conclude that using an ultrasound guide may decrease complications [69]. Anaesthesiologists should also be cautious concerning patients with pre-existing comorbidities, such as peripheral vascular disease and diabetes mellitus, which may present subclinical neuropathies that could predispose the patient to neurological deficits following spinal anaesthesia [71].

http://dx.doi.org/10.5772/58817

Skin antiseptics like chlorhexidine have proven to be superior to iodopovidone-based solutions. ASRA advises using chlorhexidine in an alcohol solution prior to all regional anaesthetic interventions to prevent infectious complications [72]. In a recent retrospective study, the neurological complication rate when using chlorhexidine was found to be similar to the findings of other surveys [57]. However, using chlorhexidine is not entirely devoid of risk. In an editorial, Bogod [73] published two cases of chlorhexidine inducing permanent neurological injury. In one case, chlorhexidine solution was inadvertently administered into the epidural space. In the second case, 0. 1 mL anticeptic of solution (chlorhexidine) mixed with a local anaesthetic was wrongly administered to the subarachnoid space. The author advised using a spray formulation for skin preparation, warning against high concentrations [more than 2%]. Applying one puff was concluded to be sufficient and emphasize was placed on waiting for the skin to dry.

Figure 2 shows medullaris cone injury secondary to attempted spinal anaesthesia in an obstetric patient undergoing a caesarean section. This patient had severe pain during bupivacaine injection. The injury was managed with steroids. Final neurological damage was minimal.

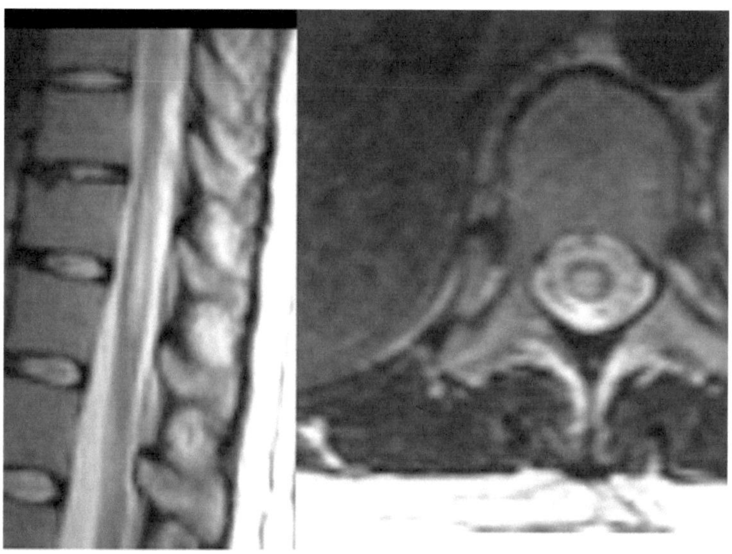

Figure 2. Sagittal and axial images of the conus medullaris T2 weighted FSE in which a high signal is noted at the centre position, with conus oedema and/or haemorrhage caused by a spinal needle (Source: www. anestesia-dolor. org).

10. Neurological diseases

Patients with pre-existing neurological diseases such as multiple sclerosis, amyotrophic lateral sclerosis, or a post-poliomyelitis condition have previously been considered as relative contraindications for neuraxial anaesthesia. A double crush phenomenon was described to explain the deterioration of neurological disease in the case of vulnerable neurons. It is believed that mechanical trauma caused by a needle or catheter, toxicity induced by local anaesthetics or neural ischaemia due to additives could worsen the patient's neurological status. Increased stress may induce inflammation deteriorates the clinical course, that may confuse with neural injury due to the procedure. However, recent evidence has demonstrated that spinal anaesthesia might be an option in this patient group [72].

Neuraxial anaesthesia in patients with spinal canal pathology, including lumbar disk disease, spinal stenosis or previous surgery, is another issue that requires special concern. In a retrospective review, Hebl et al. [74] found that patients with pre-existing spinal canal pathology demonstrated a higher rate of neurological complications. However, a lack of control groups receiving general anaesthesia presents a difficulty for describing results pertaining to whether complications occur due to surgery or because of the natural progression of disease. Additionally, due to data combinations, it is also impossible to conclude the particular role of single shot spinal anaesthesia. Trauma and complications may be more common when using large gauge Tuohy needles, or during catheter placement. Epidural anaesthesia and catheter placement in patients with previous spinal surgery appear to be more complicated, even when performed by experienced hands [75]. These patients require special attention in terms of evaluating the use of neuraxial anaesthesia, preoperative neurological evaluation and special care in order to prevent additional injuries.

In rare instances, silent pathologies involving the spinal column may induce acute postoperative neurological complications such as tuberculosis [76] or unrecognized spinal tumour [77]. Patients with coexisting or previous low back pain and paraesthesia or neurologic deficits should be carefully assessed preoperatively and their evaluation should include a detailed neurologic examination and radiological images. Moreover, patients with neural tube defects should be assessed earlier to determine the conus medullaris level or other possible associated anomalies to decide whether neuraxial techniques will provide them with safe anaesthetic options.

Patients like those described above are at higher risk of neurological complications than the rest of the general population [78]. Postoperative neurological complications were observed in a patient presenting adhesive arachnoiditis, extensive syringomyelia and a giant arachnoid cyst in the patient had been managed with a combination of spinal and epidural anaesthesia. These rare complications were linked to a reaction caused by the subarachnoid, the epidural drug, or as a result of catheter induced inflammation or trauma [79].

The images in Figure 3 show a case of multiple neurofibromatosis with intrathecal participation, which was managed with uncomplicated spinal anaesthesia.

http://dx.doi.org/10.5772/58817

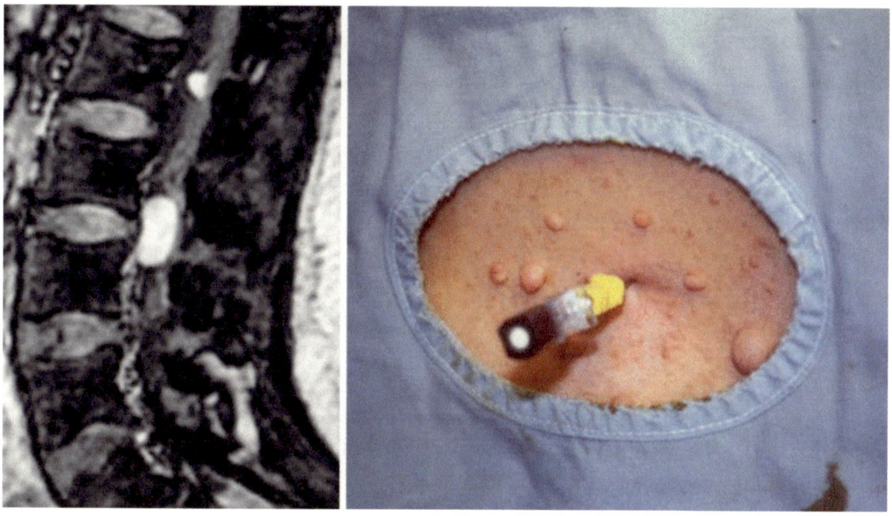

Figure 3. Forty-year-old patient with multiple neurofibromatosis. She was anesthetized successfully with spinal anaesthesia for an abdominal hysterectomy. The back of the patient shows numerous skin tumours and some cafe au lait spots. The sagittal image of the lumbar spine in post-spin echo fat-suppressed contrast demonstrates intradural solid tumours in cauda equina nerves (Source: www. anestesia-dolor. org).

11. Cardiac arrest and perioperative death

Bradycardia and cardiac arrest are the most worrisome complications related to spinal anaesthesia. The incidence of these conditions has been observed to be higher with spinal block in comparison with general anaesthesia. Patients are generally healthy, ASA class I or II, athletic and male with parasympathetic overtones. The influence of cardio-accelerator fibres originating between T1 to T4 plays a crucial role in maintaining blood pressure and heart rate according to the level of anaesthesia induced by spinal block, depleted vascular volume or insufficient replacement with fluids, and the presence of deep sedation is considered a risk factors for bradycardia and cardiac arrest. Surgical intervention may also trigger bradycardia and cardiac arrest by vagal discharge or embolization. In the case of severe bradycardia, early administration of epinephrine is important, especially in unresponsive cases to atropine and ephedrine that should be administered previously [80]. Most patients are monitored in the operating theatre, therefore early recognition of bradicardia and cardiac arrest and intervention is possible. Survival rate is higher in patients with cardiac arrest observed during spinal anaesthesia compared to cases using general anaesthesia. [81]. A study by Chatzmichali and colleagues [82] showed that assessment of heart rate variability in the preoperative period may help to determine perioperative severe bradycardia. Clinicians must be cautious when performing deep intravenous sedation, especially in patients with increased body weight, since it may lead to death in the early postoperative period.

12. Miscellaneous complications

Myoclonus occurs rarely as a complication of spinal anaesthesia in the postoperative period. It may commonly be observed in the presence of systemic illness, drug use or with a pre-existing vitamin B deficiency. Although the underlying mechanism for myoclonus in this instance is unclear, the possibility of subclinical neuropathy has been mentioned [83]. Long-term treatment, including neuroleptics and benzodiazepines, might be required to relieve the symptoms of myoclonus [83].

Exposure to the halogenated compounds during general anaesthesia is an interesting topic, especially in the context of the brain, which is currently under development as it relates to aged patients. Spinal anaesthesia appears to be safe for preventing postoperative delirium and cognitive dysfunction in the elderly, especially when additional measurements such as early pain management, supplemental oxygen, fluid, caloric replacement and morphine avoidance are applied [84].

Table 1 is a summary of the complications of neuraxial anaesthesia found in Finland. The authors reported 1:17 741 spinal block cases and 1:24 285 cases of epidural blocks. Complications were more severe in the application of spinal anaesthesia.

Claim motive	Spinal	Epidural	Total
Cardiac arrest	2 [2]	0	2
Neurological	31 [19]	7 [4]	38
Infectious	4 [4]	6 [2]	10
Local anaesthetics acute toxicity	0	2 [2]	2
Opioid overdose	0	1 [1]	1
PDPH	9	8	17
Others	13	3	16
Patients who died or contracted permanent neuronal damage are shown in parentheses			

Table 1. Severe complications associated with epidural and spinal anaesthesia [85].

13. Conclusions

Various complications may occur during spinal anaesthesia and are widely related to the procedure itself or drugs used during the procedure. These complications occur with differing incidence and in the case of at least some, appear to be inevitable and to be expected due to the invasive nature of the blockade.

Many of these complications can be reduced with meticulous attention to the details during the performance of the spinal block. The procedure may be rendered more patient-oriented and convenient by selecting the appropriate technique, drugs and their doses. It is of prime importance that the incidence of hypotension should be decreased, as this can induce serious adverse outcomes. Ultrasound guides may be helpful for decreasing complications in difficult cases. In order to decrease serious complications, patient selection and adherence to the guidelines appears to be fundamental. (such as patients with previous lumbar surgery as mentioned)

Author details

Alparslan Apan and Özgün Cuvaş Apan

Giresun University Faculty of Medicine Department of Anaesthesiology and Intensive Care Medicine , Giresun, Turkey

References

[1] Cook TM, Counsell D, Wildsmith JAW. Major complication of central neuraxial block: report on the third national audit project of the Royal College of Anaesthetists. Br J Anaesth. 2009;102:79-90.

[2] Jeon YT, Hwang JW, Kim MH, Oh AY, Park KH, Park HP, Lee Y, Do SH. Positional blood pressure change and the risk of hypotension during spinal anesthesia for cesarean delivery. Anesth Analg. 2010;111:712-5.

[3] Zorko N, Kamenik M, Starc V. The effect of Trendelenburg position, lactated ringer's solution and hydroxyethyl starch solution on cardiac output after spinal anesthesia. Anesth Analg. 2009;108:655-9.

[4] Shin BS, Kim CS, Sim WS, et al. A comparison of the effects of preanesthetic administration of crystalloid versus colloid on intrathecal spread of isobaric spinal anesthetics and cerebrospinal fluid movement. Anesth Analg. 2011;112:924-30.

[5] Hwang JW, Oh AY, Song IA, Na HS, Ry JH, Park HP, Jeon YT, Do SH. Influence of prolonged lateral position in induction of spinal anesthesia for cesarean delivery: a randomized controlled trial. Minerva Anestesiol. 2012;78:646-52.

[6] Sharwood-Smith G, Drummond GB. Hypotension in obstetric spinal anaesthesia: a lesson from pre-eclampsia. Br J Anaesth. 2009;102:291-4.

[7] Nygan Kee WD, Khaw KS, Lau TK, Ng FF, Choi K, Ng KL. Randomized double-blinded comparison of phenylephrine vs. ephedrine for maintaining blood pressure during spinal anaesthesia for non-elective Caesarean section. Anaesthesia. 2008;63:1319-26.

[8] Langesaeter E, Dyer RA. Maternal haemodynamic changes during spinal anesthesia for caesarean section. Curr Opin Anesthesiol. 2011;24:242-8.

[9] Nygan Kee WD, Khaw KS, Ng FF, Lee BB. Prophylactic phenylephrine infusion for preventing hypotension during spinal anesthesia for cesarean delivery. Anesth Analg. 2004;98:815-21.

[10] Crowley LJ, Buggy DJ. Shivering and neuraxial anesthesia. Reg Anesth Pain Med. 2008;33:241-52.

[11] Bezov D, Lipton RB, Ashina S. Post-dural puncture headache: part I diagnosis, epidemiology, etiology, and pathophysiology. Headache. 2010;50:1144-52.

[12] Lomax S, Qureshi A. Unusually early onset of post-dural puncture headache after spinal anaesthesia using a 27 g Whitacre needle. Br J Anaesth. 2008;100:707-8.

[13] Hendricks M, Stocks GM. Post-dural puncture headache in the parturient. Anaesth Intensive Care Med. 2007;8:309-11.

[14] Douglas MJ, Ward ME, Campbell DC, Bright SB, Merrik PM. Factors involved in the incidence of postdural puncture headache with 25 gauge Whitacre needle for obstetric anesthesia. Int J Obstet Anesth. 1997;6:220-3.

[15] Satanen U, Rautoma P, Luurila H, et al. Comparison of 27 gauge Whitacre and Quincke spinal needles with respect to postdural puncture headache and non-dural puncture headache. Acta Anaesthesiol Scand. 2004;48:474-9.

[16] Schmittner MD, Terboven T, Dluzak M, Janke A, Limmer ME, Weiss C, Bussen DG, Burmeister MA, Beck GC. High incidence of post-dural puncture headache in patients with spinal saddle block induced with Quincke needles for anorectal surgery: a randomized clinical trial. Int J Colorectal Dis. 2010;25:775-81.

[17] Van Der Velde M, Schepers R, Berends N, Vandermeersh E, De Buck F. Ten years of experience with accidental dural puncture headache in a tertiary anaesthesia department. Int J Obstet Anesth. 2009;17:329-35.

[18] Velickovic IA, Rostislav P. Pneumocephalus complicated by postdural puncture headache for unintentional dural puncture. Anesth Analg. 2007;104:747-8.

[19] Al-metwalli RR. Epidural morphine injections for preventing of post dural puncture headache. Anaesthesia. 2008;67:847-50.

[20] Kawaguchi M, Hashizume K, Watanabe K, Inoue S, Furuya H. Fluoroscopically guided epidural blood patch in patients with postdural puncture headache after spinal and epidural anesthesia. J Anesth. 2011;25:450-3.

[21] Boyle JAH, Stocks GM. Post-dural puncture headache in the parturient an update. Anaesth Intensive Care Med. 2010;11:302-4.

[22] Schievink WI, Maya MM, Moser FM. Treatment of spontaneous intracranial hypotension with percutaneous placement of fibrin sealant: report of four cases. J Neurosurg. 2004;100:1098-100.

[23] Schievink WI, Morreale VM, Atkinson JL, Meyer FB, Piepgras DS, Ebersold MJ. Surgical treatment of spontaneous spinal cerebrospinal fluid leaks. J Neurosurg. 1998;88:243-6.

[24] Zeidan A, Chaaban M, Farhat O, Barka A. Cerebral rebleeding by spinal anesthesia in a patient with undiagnosed chronic subdural hematoma. Anesthesiology. 2006;104;613-4.

[25] Lam DH. Subarachnoid haematoma after spinal anaesthesia mimicking transient radicular irritation: a case report and review. Anaesthesia. 2008;63:423-7.

[26] Arcand G, Girard T, McCormack M, Chouinard P, Boudreault D, Williams S. Bilateral sixth cranial nerve palsy after unintentional dural puncture. Can J Anaesth. 2004;51:821-3.

[27] Fang JY, Lin JW, Li Q, Jiang N, Gao Y. Trigeminal nerve and facial nerve palsy after combined spinal-epidural anesthesia for cesarean section. J Clin Anesth. 2010;22:56-8.

[28] Ho CM, Chan KH. Posterior reversible encephalopathy syndrome with vasospasm in a postpartum woman after postdural puncture headache following spinal anesthesia. Anesth Analg. 2007;105:770-2.

[29] Takeuchi S, Nagatani K, Otani N, Nawashino H. PRES after spinal anesthesia. J Headache Pain. 2011;12:389.

[30] Malhotra SK, Iyer BA, Gupta AK, Raghunatan M, Nakra D. Spinal analgesia and auditory functions: a comparison of two sizes of Quincke needle. Minerva Anestesiol. 2007;73:395-9.

[31] Yildiz TS, Solak M, Iseri M, Karaca B, Toker K. Hearing loss after spinal anesthesia: the effect of different solutions. Otolaryngol Head Neck Surg. 2007;137:79-82.

[32] Enron S, Gurstieva V, Ezri T, Gladkov V, Shopin S, Herman A, Sidi A, Weitzman S. Transient neurologic symptoms after isobaric subarachnoid anesthesia with 2% lidocaine: the impact of needle type. Anesth Analg. 2007;105:1494-9.

[33] Zaric D, Christiansen C, Pace NL, Punjaswadwong Y. Transient neurologic symptoms after spinal anesthesia with lidocaine versus other local anesthetic: systematic review of randomized, controlled trial. Anesth Analg. 2005;100:1811-6.

[34] Karason S, Olafsson TA. Avoiding bladder catheterization in total knee arthroplasty: patient selection criteria and low dose spinal anesthesia. Acta Anaesthesiol Scand. 2013;57:639-45.

[35] Kamphuis ET, Kuipers PW, van Venrooij GE, Kalkman CJ. The effects of spinal anesthesia with lidocaine and sufentanil on lower urinary tract functions. Anesth Analg. 2008;107:2073-8.

[36] Kamphuis ET, Ionescu TI, Kuipers PWG, de Gier J, van Venrooij GEMP, Boon TA. Recovery of storage and emptying functions of the bladder after spinal anesthesia with lidocaine and with bupivacaine in men. Anesthesiology. 1998;88:310-6.

[37] Lau H, Lam B. Management of postoperative urinary retention. A randomized trial of in-out versus overnight catheterization. ANZ J Surg. 2004;74:658-61.

[38] Keita H, Diouf E, Tubach F, Brouwer T, Dahmani S, Mantz J, Desmonts JM. Predictive factors of early postoperative urinary retention in the postanesthesia care unit. Anesth Analg. 2005;101:592-6.

[39] Dreijer B, Møller MH, Barthody J. Post-operative urinary retention in a general surgical populations. Eur J Anaesthesiol. 2011;28:190-4.

[40] Pöpping DM, Elia N, Marret E, Wenk M, Tramèr MR. Opioids added to local anesthetics for single-shot intrathecal anesthesia in patients undergoing minor surgery: a meta-analysis of randomized trials. Pain. 2012;153:784-93.

[41] Choi S, Mahon P. Neuroaxial anesthesia and bladder dysfunction in the perioperative period: a systematic review. Can J Anaesth. 2012;59:681-703.

[42] Kawamata YT, Nishikawa K, Kawamata T, Omote K, Igarashi M, Yamauchi M, Sato K, Nakayama M, Namiki A. A comparison of hyperbaric 1% and 3% solutions of small-dose lidocaine in spinal anesthesia. Anesth Analg. 2003;96:881-4.

[43] Baldini G, Bagry A, Aprikian A, Carli F. Postoperative urinary retention. Anesthesiology. 2009;110:1139-57.

[44] Lamonerie L, Marret E, Deleuze A, Lembert N, Dupont M, Bonnet F. Prevalence of postoperative bladder distention and urinary retention detected by ultrasound measurements. Br J Anaesth. 2004;92:544-6.

[45] Horlocker TT. Regional anaesthesia in the patient receiving antithrombotic and antiplatelet therapy. Br J Anaesth. 2011;107:i96-i106. (no)

[46] Moen V, Dahlgren N, Irestedt L. Severe neurological complications after central neuraxial blockades in Sweden 1990-1999. Anesthesiology. 2004;101:950-9.

[47] Horlocker TT, Wedel DJ, Rowlingson JC, Enneking FK, Kopp SL, Benzon HT, Brown DL, Heit JA, Mulroy MF, Rosenquist RW, Tryba M, Yuan CS. Regional anesthesia in the patient receiving antithrombotic or thrombolytic therapy: American Society of Regional Anesthesia and Pain Medicine evidence-based guidelines. Reg Anesth Pain Med. 2010;35:64-101.

[48] Gogarten W, Vandermeulen E, Van Aken H, Kozek S, Llau JV, Samma CM. Regional anaesthesia and antithrombotic agents: recommendations of the European Society of Anaesthesiology. Eur J Anaesthesiol. 2010;27:999-1015.

[49] Breivik H, Bang U, Jalonen J, Vigfùsson G, Alahuhta S, Lagerranser M. Nordic guideline for neuraxial blocks in disturbed haemostasis from the Scandinavian Society of Anaesthesiology and Intensive Care Medicine. Acta Anaesthesiol Scand. 2010;54:16-41.

[50] Choi S, Brull R. Neuraxial techniques in obstetric and non-obstetric patients with common bleeding diatheses. Anesth Analg. 2009;109:648-60.

[51] Van Veen JJ, Nokes TJ, Makris M. The risk of spinal haematoma following neuraxial anaesthesia or lumbar puncture in thrombocytopenic individuals. Br J Hematol. 2009;148:15-25.

[52] Schulz-Stübner S, Pottinger JM, Coffin SA, Herwaldt LA. Nosocomial infections and infection control in regional anesthesia. Acta Anaesthesiol Scand. 2008;52:1144-57.

[53] Baer ET. Post-dural puncture bacterial meningitis. Anesthesiology. 2006;105:381-93.

[54] Gritsenko K, Marcello D, Liguori GA, Jules-Elysèe K, Memtsoudis SG. Meningitis or epidural abscesses after neuraxial block for removal of infected hip or knee prosthesis. Br J Anaesth. 2012;108:485-90.

[55] Bader AM, Gilbertson L, Kirz L, Datta S. Regional anesthesia in woman with chorioamnionitis. Reg Anesth. 1992;17:84-6.

[56] Goodman EJ, DeHorta E, Taguiam JM. Safety of spinal and epidural anesthesia in parturients with chorioamnionitis. Reg Anesth Pain Med. 1996;21:436-41.

[57] Sviggum HP, Jacop AK, Arendt KW, Mauermann ML, Horlocker TT, Hebl JR. Neurologic complications after chlorhexidine antisepsis for spinal anesthesia. Reg Anesth Pain Med. 2012;37:139-44.

[58] Tsai PS, Hsu CS, Fan YC, Huang CJ. General anaesthesia is associated with increased risk of surgical site infection after caesarean delivery compared with neuraxial anaesthesia: a population-based study. Br J Anaesth. 2011; 21:275-80.

[59] Brull R, McCartney CJ, Chan VW, El-Beheiry H. Neurological complications after regional anesthesia: contemporary estimates of risk. Anesth Analg. 2007;104:965-74.

[60] Hebl JR. The importance and implications of aseptic techniques during regional anesthesia. Reg Anesth Pain Med. 2006;31:311-23.

[61] de Sèze MP, Sztark F, Janvier G, Joseph PA. Severe and long-lasting complications of the nerve root and spinal cord central neuraxial blockade. Anesth Analg 2007;104:975-9.

[62] Ko JY, Leffert LR. Clinical implications of neuraxial anesthesia in the parturient with scoliosis. Anesth Analg. 2009;109:1930-4.

[63] Horlocker TT. Complication of regional anesthesia and acute pain management. Anesthesiol Clin. 2011;29:257-78.

[64] Reynolds F. Damage to the conus medullaris following spinal anaesthesia. Anaesthesia. 2001;56:238-47.

[65] Broadbent CR, Maxwell WB, Ferrie R, Wilson DJ, Gawne-Cain M, Russel R. Ability of anaesthetists to identify a marked lumbar interspace. Anaesthesia 2000;55:1122-6.

[66] Furnes G, Reilly MP, Kuchi S. An evaluation of ultrasound imaging for identification of lumbar intervertebral level. Anaesthesia. 2002;57:277-80.

[67] Kim JT, Bahk JH, Sung T. Influence of age and sex on the position of the conus medullaris and Tuffier's line in adults. Anesthesiology. 2003;99:1359-63.

[68] Lin N, Bebawy JF, Hua L, Wang BG. Is spinal anaesthesia at L2-L3 interspace safe in disorders of the vertebral column? A magnetic resonance imaging study. Br J Anaesth. 2010;105:857-62.

[69] Neal JM, Bernards CM, Hadzic A, Hebl JR, Hogan QH, Horlocker TT, Lee LA, Rathmell JP, Sorenson EJ, Suresh S, Wedel DJ. ASRA practice advisory on neurologic complications in regional anesthesia and pain medicine. Reg Anesth Pain Med. 2008;33:404-15.

[70] Chin KJ, Perlas A, Chan V, Brown-Shreves D, Koshkin A, Vaishnav V. Ultrasound imaging facilitates spinal anesthesia in adults with difficult surface anatomic landmarks. Anesthesiology. 2011;105:94-101.

[71] Angadi DS, Garde A. Subclinical neuropathy in diabetic patients: a risk factor for bilateral lower limb neurological deficit following spinal anesthesia? J Anesth. 2012;26:107-10.

[72] Hebl JR, Horlocker TT, Schroeder DR. Neuraxial anesthesia and analgesia in patients with preexisting central nervous system disorder. Anesth Analg. 2006;103:223-8.

[73] Bogod D. The sting in the tail: antiseptics and the neuraxis revisited. Anaesthesia. 2012;67:1305-9.

[74] Hebl JR, Horlocker TT, Kopp SL, Schroeder DR. Neuraxial blockade in patients with preexisting spinal stenosis, lumbar disk disease, or prior spine surgery: efficacy and neurologic complications. Anesth Analg. 2010;111:1511-9.

[75] Daley MD, Rolbin SH, Hew EM, Morningstar BA, Stewart JA. Epidural anesthesia for obstetrics after spinal surgery. Reg Anesth. 1990;15:280-4.

[76] Karaaslan P, Candan S, Basaran C. Paraplegia after spinal anesthesia as a result of previous undiagnosed vertebral tuberculosis. Anesth Analg. 2006;102:1300-1.

[77] Cerroni A, Carvalho JA, Tancredi A, Volpe AR, Floccare A. Acute bleeding after spinal anesthesia due to puncture of unsuspected lumbar myxopependimoma. Eur J Anaesthesiol. 2010;27:1072-4.

[78] Valente A, Frassanito L, Natale L, Draisci G. Occult spinal dysraphism in obstetric: a case of caesarean section with subarachnoid anaesthesia after remifentanil intravenous analgesia for labour. Case reports in Obstet Gynecol. 2012;472482:1-3.

[79] Hirai T, Kato T, Kawabata S, Enomoto M, Tomizawa S, Yoshi T, Sakaki K, Shinomiya, Okawa A. Adhesive arachnoiditis with extensive syringomyelia and giant arachnoid cyst after spinal and epidural anesthesia. Spine. 2012;237: E195-E198.

[80] Limongi JAG, de Melo Lins RSA. Cardiopulmonary arrest in spinal anesthesia. Rev Bras Anestesiol. 2011;61:110-20.

[81] Kopp SL, Horlocker TT, Warner ME, Hebl JR, Vachon CA, Schroeder DR, Gould AB Sprung V. Cardiac arrest during neuraxial anesthesia: frequency and predisposing factors. Anesth Analg. 2005;100: 855-65.

[82] Chatzimichali A, Zoumprouli A, Metaxari M, Apostolakis I, Daras T, Tzanakis N, Askitopoulou H. Hearth rate variability may identify patients who will develop severe bradycardia during spinal anaesthesia. Acta Anaesthesiol Scand. 2010;55:234-41.

[83] Menezes FV, Venkat N. Spinal myoclonus following combined spinal-epidural anesthesia for cesarean section. Anaesthesia. 2006;61:597-600.

[84] Björkelund KB, Hommel A, Thorgren KG, Gustafson L, Larsson S, Lundberg D. Reducing delirium in elderly patients with hip fracture: a multi-factorial intervention study. Acta Anaesthesiol Scand. 2010;54:678-88.

[85] Aromaa U, Lahdensuu M, Cozanitis DA. Severe complications associated with epidural and spinal anaesthesia in Finland 1987-1993. A study based on patient insurance claims. Acta Anaesthesiol Scand. 1997;41:445-452.

Chapter 8

Spinal or Epidural Haematoma

R. Hakan Erbay, Nimet Senoglu and Habip Atalay

Additional information is available at the end of the chapter

http://dx.doi.org/10.5772/58702

1. Introduction

Intravertebral haematomas may occur in the epidural or subdural space. Generally speaking all intravertebral haematomas are also referred as "spinal haematomas". It is an infrequently described complication of neuroaxial anaesthesia techniques. It has been described in the literature in patients with a deranged coagulation profile in the form of systemic diseases (e.g. chronic renal failure, liver failure) or anticoagulant therapy. In this chapter we will discuss spinal haematomas as a devastating complication of the neuroaxial anaesthesia techniques.

2. Etiopathogenesis of spinal haematoma

Spinal haematoma is the accumulation of blood in the potential space between the dura and bone. It can be a complication of neuroaxial anaesthesia techniques, especially in those patients with a deranged coagulation profile due to systemic diseases (e.g. hepatic diseases, renal failure) or anticoagulant therapy. It is more common in the patients treated with anticoagulants, thrombocytopenia, or in patients with alcoholic liver disease.

Advanced liver disease, with associated portal hypertension and hypersplenism, thrombocytopenia, platelet dysfunction, reduced production of clotting factors, increased clotting factor consumption, and increased fibrinolysis may also increase the risk of bleeding. Before neuroaxial anaesthesia is planned, it is very important to detect liver diseases. The laboratory tests needed are; haemoglobin, PT, aPTT, INR, platelet count, platelet function analysis, and fibrinogen level. Dunn et al. reported that in a case with renal disease also causes haemostatic defects due to defects in platelets, subendothelial metabolism, and platelet vessel interactions. The metabolism of antiplatelet drugs and low-molecular-weight heparins is also reduced during kidney failure. Coagulation profile tests; bleeding time, PT, PTT, must be performed in all patients with renal failure. Grejda and colleagues reported a case with clotting abnormalities, apparently due to chronic renal failure, who developed paraplegia after spinal anaesthesia secondary to spinal hematoma formation [1, 2].

Malnutrition, fat malabsorption, antibiotic usage, and liver disease may be cause for vitamin k deficiency. Vitamin k deficit leads to a reduction of microsomal carboxylase, a liver enzyme dependent on vitamin k activity, which induce lack of converting factors II, VII, IX, and X into their functionally active forms and consequently, a bleeding diathesis. The clinical findings in these patients are melena, hematuria, ecchymoses and haematomas. In the patient at-risk of bleeding it is recommended to give vitamin k supplements hours prior to a procedure [3].

Other considered factors favouring the formation of a spinal haematoma include: trauma, thrombolysis, lumbar puncture, disc herniation and the vertebral procedures, epidural or spinal anaesthesia, coagulopathy or bleeding diathesis, hepatic disease with portal hypertension, and vascular malformations. Less common causes include systemic lupus erythematosus, ankylosing spondylitis, rheumatoid arthritis, Paget's disease in vertebral bones, Valsalva manoeuvre and hypertension. In 40 to 50% of spinal haematomas there was not an apparent underlying cause [4].

The haemorrhage into the spinal canal frequently occurs in the epidural space due to epidural venous plexus rupture (Baston venous plexus), however arterial haemorrhage may also occur [5, 6]. Nevertheless, the main source of bleeding (arterial or venous) is controversial. Spinal haematoma can be seen quickly with arterial bleeding and can lead to neural trauma and ischemia. However, when aetiology is the needle or the epidural catheter, the spinal haematoma may become symptomatic after a few days, so this situation suggests that the cause is not arterial bleeding. Therefore, spinal haematomas are mostly venous because there are no valves in the epidural venous plexus and the pressure in the epidural space is low. Venous plexus blood flow can be reversed with physical activity and the sudden increases in intra-abdominal and intrathoracic pressure (Valsalva manoeuvre). Epidural venous pressure elevation and hemodynamic changes in pregnancy can also cause rupture on the venous vessel walls. Venous bleeding accumulates slowly, but it can theoretically tamponade the epidural space before exceeding the spinal cord perfusion pressure. Thus, the whole clinical situation may not be clearly understood. The amount of blood causing cord ischemia is variable, and it depends on the speed of blood accumulation. Interestingly, most of the blood volume of the haematomas associated with low-molecular-weight heparin (LMWH) is less than the injected blood volume for epidural patch [7].

The region of spinal haematoma is often at cervical and thoracic vertebrae level, spreading throughout the thoracolumbar spine. Most of the spinal haematomas are seen at the dorsal dural sac, because it adheres to the posterior longitudinal ligament at the front of the spinal canal. Posterior or posterolateral thoracic or lumbar regions are often involved. Usually the haematoma is limited to a few vertebral level [4].

http://dx.doi.org/10.5772/58702

3. Frequency

In the current literature, the incidence of spinal haematoma is about 1/150,000 epidural anaesthesia and 1/220,000 for spinal anaesthesia [7]. From 1906 to 1994, there were 61 spinal haematoma cases reported associated with epidural or spinal anaesthesia [5]. 87% of the patients had haemostatic abnormalities, traumatic or difficult needle insertion attempt, and in 33% of these cases had more than one risk factor. What is relevant is that only 38% of patients had partial or complete neurological recovery. A retrospective study from China reviewed medical records from 1954 to 2008 and found an incidence of 2.14/100.000 (95% confidence interval: 0.44-6.25/100.000) of spinal haematomas after neuraxial blockade. The presence of bacterial infection and the need of emergency surgery were found to increase the risk of epidural haematoma. In general, the risk of major bleeding were multifactorial and increased with age (and associated with abnormalities of the spinal cord or vertebral column), the presence of coagulopathy, anticoagulation (especially standard heparin or LMWH), traumatic needle or catheter insertion. There is a correlation between early decompression surgeries with a better neurological recovery. [8] If laminectomy is performed within 8 hours after the onset of neurological dysfunctions, spinal cord ischemia tends to be reversible [9]. Spinal haematomas are responsible for about half of all spinal cord injuries [10].

The true incidence of neurological dysfunction due to hemorrhagic complications associated with neuroaxial block is not known. Importantly, postoperative numbness or weakness are typically thought to be secondary to the injected local anaesthetic, therefore the diagnosis of cord ischemia may be delayed. On the other hand, patient proper care rarely have the standard level of treatment (1/13 cases), and health care costs are very high. It is impossible to identify the exact risk factors of spinal haematomas from case series. However, the incidence of large surveillance studies (including spinal haematoma) investigated the frequency of high-and low-risk groups are identified. An epidemiological study from Sweden for a 10 years period with 1,260,000 spinal and 450,000 epidural blocks was investigated for serious neurological complications [9]. There were 33 spinal haematoma cases, and from those 24 cases were women and 25 cases were associated with epidural technique. The risk is lower in young women (for epidural analgesia, 1/200,000) than older women (for knee arthroplasty, 1/3,600). Similarly, in women, the risk of spinal haematoma with a hip fracture surgery under spinal anaesthesia (1/22,000) is higher than all spinal anaesthesia (1/480,000) [7, 9].

4. History and physical examination

Needle placement into the spinal or epidural space may damage an epidural vein or artery and causes spinal haematoma formation. Irritation of nerve roots in the epidural space results in acute back pain, and may also cause spinal compression. Impairing vibration, two point discrimination, and position sense are the first clinical findings because the posterior spinal columns are the first structure to be affected. If the cortical spinal motor tracts are compromised resulting from expanded haematoma, the patient becomes paraplegic. The last clinical findings are pain, temperature changes, and light touch alterations because the anterior lateral spinal thalamic tract is the last structure to be affected [11].

The patient is usually very disturbed, and has often severe, localized and constant low back pain. In addition, a radicular component mimicking disc herniation can be seen. Weakness, drowsiness, urinary or faecal incontinence may be accompanied. In most cases, pain starts spontaneously, but sometimes pain can be associated with minor symptoms such as defecation, lifting, coughing and sneezing. Spinal cord and nerve root dysfunction, depending on the level of the lesion develops quickly and rapidly progression to paraparesis or paraplegia. Low back pain increases with increasing intraspinal pressure manoeuvres that stretching along the spine such as cough, sneeze and percussion. Depending on the size and location of the spinal haematoma the physical findings includes unilateral or bilateral weakness, sensory loss with unilateral or bilateral radicular paresthesia, deep tendon reflexes in the form of various modifications and changes in the bladder and anal sphincter tone.

Lumbar epidural haematoma may mimic an acute disc herniation. Epidural haematoma due to neuroaxial anaesthesia or lumbar puncture may represent new or progressive postoperative neurological symptoms. A time delay in return of loss of sensory or motor (with or without back pain) function after spinal or epidural block, are pathognomonic signals of spinal haematoma, and until proven otherwise, treatment should be considered [4].

5. Diagnosis

Spinal epidural haematoma is usually diagnosed based on the acute neurological deficits, a rapid loss of motor and sensorial function, paraplegia, quadriplegia, or autonomic dysfunction. Quite often patients have acute radiating pain, sensory nerve root or spinal cord compression and focal neurologic deficit. Postoperative epidural haematoma is usually seen in the first 24-48 hours after the neuraxial block. Back pain and lower limb weakness as well as sensory deficit should alert the clinician to the presence of a central compressing lesion. Early clinical signs of pain or focal neurologic deficit are found in the postoperative period. Any new or progressive neurological symptoms or bowel and bladder incontinence require rapid clinical evaluation and diagnostic studies. If a new or progressive neurologic deficit is observed during epidural analgesia infusion, this requires an immediate discontinuation. The epidural catheter is left in place, and no more local anaesthetics are injected because of an early warning signs may be masked by their injection. If an epidural infusion causes the neurological findings, the return of sensory and motor function should be noted when the local anaesthetic effect wear off. On the other hand, speedy radiographic imaging studies and a neurosurgical consultation should be carried out. If there is an acute neurological deficit with low back pain, nerve root and spinal cord compression. An urgent assessment should be made to distinguish situations that mimic spinal haematoma such as epidural abscess, spinal cord disease,

http://dx.doi.org/10.5772/58702

neoplasia, and acute herniated disc. Also, new or progressive neurological manifestations includes muscular or ligamentous injury related to needle placement, postoperative surgical neuropraxia, prolonged or exaggerated neuroaxial block, anterior spinal artery syndrome, and pre-existing undiagnosed neurological disorder need to be discarded.

Complete blood counts including platelets should be done, and the presence of infection should be investigated. Prothrombin time, aPTT, and INR are very useful to study bleeding diathesis

Urgent radiographic diagnostic studies are essential to avoid delay in surgical treatment of spinal haematomas. Magnetic resonance imaging (MRI) is the preferred method due to the rapid and non-invasive technique. MRI can detect presence of the spinal haematoma and location of associated vascular malformation; define the degree of compression of the cord. Also, the age of the haematoma can be diagnosed by MRI. Chronological MRI characteristics of spinal haematoma are similar to intracranial haemorrhage. In hyper acute period (first 6 hours), presence of spinal haematoma is seen isointense in T1-weighted images and mildly hyperintense and heterogeneity in T2-weighted images. In acute period (7-72 hours) hematoma is still isointense on T1-weighted images and begin to hypointense on T2-weighted images. This depends on intracellular deoxyhemoglobine and T2 becomes shorter. With the increase in the concentration of metahemoglobin, haematoma T1 and T2 hyperintense also starts to become homogeneous [4]. (Figure 1).

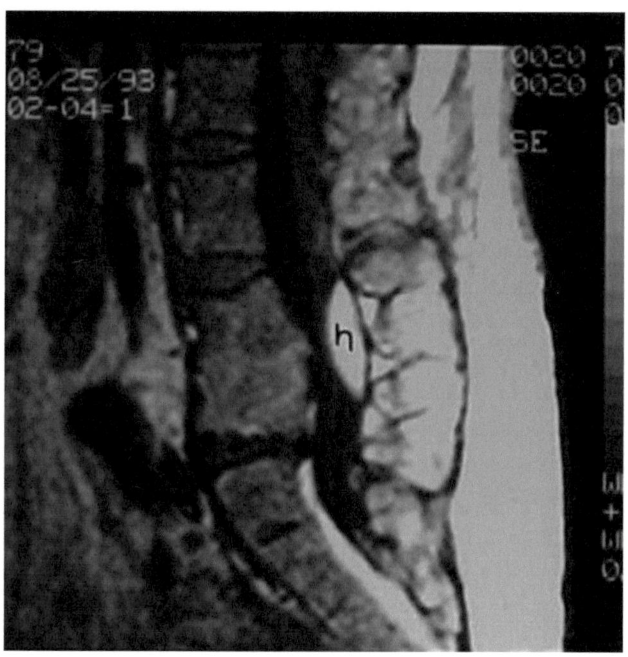

Figure 1. Sagital T1 MRI showing an epidural haematoma (h) due to an epidural block in an anticoagulated patient. Courtesy of www.anestesia-dolor.org

Epidural haematoma may be diagnosed by conventional CT, but if the thecal sac or spinal cord haematoma is isodense and if the upper thoracic region image quality is affected by artefacts the result may falsely negative. Also, CT may not be diagnostic for thoracic spinal level because the resolution is high contrast between the vertebral bone area and lung parenchyma.

Conventional angiography may be required to demonstrate a vascular malformation. Myelography and CT were used in the diagnosis of epidural hematomas, but they are not specific, invasive, and can worsen the clinical condition [4].

6. Precautions, treatment and prognosis

Neuraxial anaesthesia should be avoided in patients who are receiving anticoagulants drugs, patients suspected of bleeding diathesis, thrombolysis or after recent lumbar puncture. Anaesthesiologists should be constantly up to date regarding information on anticoagulation protocols, new anticoagulant medications and the guidelines for regional anaesthesia in this clinical scenario. Antithrombotic therapy in patients receiving neuroaxial block and/ or catheter removal needs special timing for the procedure. It should be based on patient regional anaesthesia benefit ratio versus risk of spinal haematoma.

Although some case reports mention that patients with epidural haematoma had been treated successfully with conservative methods, the treatment protocol should be decompressive surgery [12, 13]. Successful non operative treatment has been reported mainly at the level of the cauda equina and in patients with mild neurological symptoms. Most reports of spinal haematomas with neurologic symptoms improved when they were treated with immediate laminectomy; however, the decision of surgery belongs to the neurosurgeon. The most important factors for neurological recovery after a spinal haematoma are preoperative neurological deficit and operative interval. Neurological outcome is related to the time between clinical symptoms and surgical decompression. Early recognition is needed. The clinical symptoms are back pain (radicular), bladder dysfunction and sensory and, more often, motor deficits. These symptoms should initiate immediate further diagnostic efforts. Magnetic resonance imaging is the most appropriate tool. If transport of the patient to a hospital with MRI would prolong the start of surgical therapy considerably, other diagnostic means such as myelography or computed tomography should be considered. Immediate surgical decompression in the case of epidural haematoma is the best way to achieve neurological restitution. Most of the patients with good recovery had less than eight hours delay from the onset of symptoms to surgery [14].

If surgery is delayed, prognosis is poor [15]. For a full neurologic recovery the time interval between the onset of paralysis and surgery should not be more than 8 hours. Neurological improvement without surgery is rare, and consultation for decompression surgery should not be delayed. Overall mortality is 8%. Functional recovery is associated with the duration of symptoms, and the healing is seldom after 72 hours after symptoms have begun [16]. The prognosis for neurological recovery and neurological dysfunction primary depends on the duration of the patient's preoperative neurological status. Improvement is due to early diagnosis, hence neurological and neurosurgical consultation should be done as soon as possible. Neurological complications of spinal haematoma include paraplegia, spasticity, neuropathic pain, and urinary and anal sphincter dysfunction.

The clinician performing neuroaxial anaesthesia must be aware of the potential bleeding complication of these procedures. Most cases of spinal haematomas associated with neuroaxial anaesthesia (epidural/spinal) are related to thromboprophylaxis.The American Society of Regional Anesthesia has published guidelines addressing the risk of bleeding and haematomas following neuroaxial techniques in anticoagulated patients, cases receiving antithrombotic or thrombolytic therapy. That will be discussed in detail later in this chapter [10].

Ho et al. [17] summarized in ten steps the safety precautions to minimize the risk of spinal haematoma following epidural catheterization during cardiac surgery:

1. Normalization of coagulation before needle or catheter insertion
2. Avoidance of repeated attempts
3. Postponement of surgery for 24 hours after bloody tap
4. Needle or catheter insertion 1 hour before systemic heparinization
5. Optimization of haemostasis after cardiopulmonary bypass
6. Removal of epidural catheter only after normal haemostasis has been restored postoperatively
7. Close neurologic surveillance
8. Using midline approach technique
9. Administration of saline solution through the needle to distend the epidural space before insertion of the catheter
10. Neuroaxial instrumentation postoperatively only after normalization of coagulation.

Raj and colleagues [18] have developed a bleeding risk score, which estimated based on the potential hazards of bleeding, associated with specific anticoagulants and bleeding disorders. In this scoring system each factor count as one point; the target structure is near a major vascular or neurological structure or is in a confined space. The other factors are the calibre of the needle, the use of fluoroscopy and contrast media, and the use of aspiration are factors that influence the risk and recognition of bleeding, and a "single shot" procedure. The clinician should be made a decision to cancel or carry out the procedure according to the bleeding risk score (Table 1) and overall risk stratification (Table 2)

Risk factors associated with neuroaxial technique	**Score**
• Proximity to significant vascular structures	1
• Proximity to significant neurological structures	1
• Target in a confined space	1
• Use of a sharp, rather than blunt needle to reach target	1
• Multiple passages	1
• Contrast not used, if applicable	1
• Fluoroscopy not used, if applicable	1
• Aspiration not performed or presence of blood at needle hub	1
• Needle size larger than 20 gauge	1
• Continuous, not single shot procedure	1

Table 1. Bleeding risk score during neuroaxial blocks (adapted from reference 18)

Overall score	0-4	5-6	7-10
Overall risk stratification	Low	Medium	High

Table 2. Overall risk stratification according to the bleeding risk score

Antithrombotic therapy

In 2008 the American College of Chest Physicians (ACCP), 8th Antithrombotic and Thrombolytic Therapy Conference issued a statement [19]. Recommendations from this report are summarized in Table 3.

These recommendations have brought new challenges for the management of patients with neuraxial block. In general, the long-range high degree thromboprophylaxis is recommended. Acceptable alternative guide to ACCP is Surgical Care Improvement Project (SCIP; www.qualitynet.org). In addition, American Academy of Orthopaedic Surgeons (AAOS) has published a guide in 2007 for surgical bleeding associated with thromboprophylaxis for deep vein thrombosis in patients undergoing hip surgery to prevent pulmonary embolism (www.aaos.org / guidelines.pdf). In general, the AAOS guideline is more conservative and recommends routine mechanical prophylaxis and aggressive chemoprophylaxis in high-risk patients [10].

Understanding of mechanism of blood coagulation, pharmacological properties and clinical studies of anticoagulation and antiplatelet medication reduced the risk of spinal haematoma in neuroaxial blocks.

http://dx.doi.org/10.5772/58702

Risk level	DVT risk without thromboprophylaxis (%)*	Recommended thromboprophylaxis options
Low risk • Minor surgery in mobile patients • Medical patients who are fully mobile	<10	Not specific thromboprophylaxis Early and aggressive ambulation
Middle risk • Most of gynecological or urological patients • Internal medicine patients: in bed, middle VTE risk+high bleeding risk	10–40	DMWH (on recommended doses), LDUH or fondaparinux Mechanical thromboprophylaxis
High risk • Hip and knee arthroplasty, hip surgery • Major trauma, spinal cord injury, high VTE risk + high bleeding risk	40–80	DMWH (on recommended doses), fondaparinux, oral vitamin K antagonist (INR 2–3) Mechanical thromboprophylaxis

* Asymptomatic DVT rates with objective diagnostic screening in patients not receiving thromboprophylaxis.

† mechanical thromboprophylaxis: intermittent pneumatics pressure, venous foot pump, and/or Anti-embolism Stockings, Low molecular weight heparin (LMWH), LDUH: low dose unfractioned heparin,INR, international normalized ratio, VTE: venous thromboemboli

Table 3. The risk of thromboembolism and recommended thromboprophylaxis for patients in hospital stay [19].

7. Thrombolytic and fibrinolytic therapy

Thrombolytic agents actively dissolve the fibrin clots. Exogenous plasminogen activators (streptokinase and urokinase) are drugs used to dissolve thrombus, and also affect circulating plasminogen that is decreasing the plasminogen and fibrin levels. Recombinant tissue-type plasminogen activator (rt-PA) is more fibrin selective and has less impact on the level of circulating plasminogen. Clot lysis leads to increase the fibrin degradation products, they also inhibit platelet aggregation and has anticoagulant effect. About one day after the administration of thrombolytic agents the haemostasis is altered. Fibrinogen is the latest improved factor. In addition to fibrinolytic agent, these patients often receive intravenous heparin and clopidogrel or aspirin in order to keep 1.5-2 times higher than the normal aPTT level. There are spinal haematomas case reports in patients taking thrombolytic agents while had an epidural catheter placed [7, 9].

The contraindication guidelines for thrombolytic agents suggests that if these drugs are taken, a needle insertion attempt should not be done during the following 10 days. Although there is no precise data for a neuroaxial block attempt after stopping the drugs [7, 9].

8. Management of regional anaesthesia in patients receiving thrombolytic and fibrinolytic therapy [20].

- Patients receiving fibrinolytic or thrombolytic drugs should be considered if spinal or epidural anaesthesia are thought to be applied.
- Patients receiving fibrinolytic or thrombolytic therapy, there is no suggestion a definite time for the withdrawal of the epidural catheter. Fibrinogen level measurement may be useful to assess residual thrombolytic effect.

8.1. Oral anticoagulants

Patients have different sensitivities to anticoagulants. In very sensitive patients the effect of anticoagulants drugs is more potent and longer after their discontinuation. Prothrombin time (PT) is up to 20% higher with a single dose of 3 to 5 mg of warfarin. The patients with resistance to these drugs have shorter duration of anticoagulation. Factors that increase the sensitivity to heparin and warfarin include general medical condition, diet, > 65 years old, female gender, excessive surgical blood loss, liver, or heart, or kidney diseases [7].

Anaesthetic management of patients receiving preoperative warfarin depends on the dosage and the treatment time. In patients with chronic oral anticoagulation, PT and INR levels take 3-5 days to return to normal values after anticoagulants discontinuation. Theoretically, PT and INR will be affected more factor VII activity (factor VII half-life of 6-8 hours), the time to return to normal PT and INR, factor II and X levels may not be sufficient for haemostasis. If INR is within the normal range, vitamin k dependent factors are typically normal. Thus, the coagulation should returns to normal range before the neuraxial block [10]. Although after warfarin discontinuation PT/INR are back to normal, the residual (subclinical) warfarin anticoagulant effect may be seen postoperatively [9]. Depending on the time of warfarin initiation factor half-life: Factor VII: 6-8 hours, Factor IX: 24 hours, Factor X: 25-60 hours, Factor II: 50-80 hours.

The correlation between vitamin k dependent coagulation factors and INR should be known for the proper management of regional anaesthesia. In patients with congenital factors II, IX and X deficits, activity levels of each factor for hemostasis should be normal or at least reach to 40%. If any clotting factor level are 20-40% below of their normal values, bleeding may occur. Factor VII and X activities are sensitive to PT and INR, but factor II activity is less sensitive to them. Because factor VII have a relatively short half-life, PT and INR may increased in 24-36 hours.

When factor VII activity is approximately 55% the INR can be longer (INR > 1.2). If INR is 1.5 the activity of factor VII is about 40%. If INR is <1.5 the haemostasis should be normal. However, prolonged PT/INR with factor VII activity may range from normal to very low levels. Neuraxial catheterization is safe with normal PT/INR, but with prolonged PT/INR is difficult to interpret for VII factor activity, and as much as 10% of the epidural catheters are withdrawn early and unnecessary [6]. Adequate anaesthesia management of patients receiving warfarin has to be based on the proper knowledge of the anticoagulant pharmacology, vitamin-K-dependent factors levels, and in the experience of reported cases of spinal haematoma [10].

Proper time for withdrawal of the neuroaxial catheter is controversial. Nearly 6,000 patients who received preoperative oral anticoagulants with spinal or epidural catheters is examined with four studies [7, 21].This study showed that responses of patients with warfarin have been highly variable. Up to 48 hours after initiation of treatment PT may not be prolonged, but even after a single dose, PT prolongation occurred in significant number of patients. Larger doses (> 5 mg of warfarin) increases these findings. To avoid excessive PT prolongation, you should assess daily levels [10].

8.2. Regional anaesthesia management for the patients treated with anticoagulants [20].

- Oral anticoagulation is stopped before neuraxial block, and normalization of PT is verified.
- PT and INR are monitored daily.
- When the vitamin-K dependent factors are adequate (INR <1.5), neuraxial catheters can be pulled out.
- There is no definite recommendation when INR values are >1.5-<3.0 regarding the withdrawal of neuraxial catheters. Neurological condition should be carefully evaluated until INR stabilized, and the neuraxial catheters should be cautiously withdrawn.
- If INR > 3, warfarin should be avoided. There is no definite recommendation regarding the withdrawal of neuraxial catheters (eg. partial or complete recovery of the anticoagulant effect of warfarin, or it can be interrupt until recovery of spontaneous haemostasis).

8.3. Intravenous and subcutaneous standard (unfractionated) heparin

In high risk patients (acute thromboembolism), full systemic heparinization is given until a normal aPTT level is doubled. However, in vascular interventions, intravenous mid-level dosage of heparin (~5000 units) is given intraoperatively. Systemic heparinization in patients with spinal or epidural catheters were found to be safe in more than 4000 patients. Spinal haematomas were detected in 2% of these patients after diagnostic lumbar procedures and heparinization. In patients with anticoagulation within concomitant use of aspirin or anticoagulant therapy, after traumatic needle attempt or after a week of this attempt are defined as risk factors for spinal haematoma [7].

In general, a large number studies and clinical experience of regional anaesthesia techniques do not predict the risk of spinal haematoma during the use of systemic heparinization. However, they have stated that such events are not rare as previously thought, and if there is a suspicion for spinal haematoma diagnostic processes should be done as early as possible [10].

In patients receiving high-dose intraoperative systemic heparin, particularly in cardiac surgery. Epidural and spinal anaesthesia and analgesia has gained popularity and has not been reported cases of spinal haematomas. The possibility of epidural haematoma in these patients is for epidural anaesthesia 1/1528, and for spinal anaesthesia 1/3610 [9].

In a study conducted on 9000 patients that received subcutaneous heparin and applied spinal or epidural anaesthesia no spinal haematoma was reported. In patients receiving low-dose heparin, only four spinal haematoma has been reported after neuraxial block, epidural anaesthesia technique was applied in three of them [9]. Neuraxial block security for these patients is not known [19].

8.4. Regional anaesthesia management in patients receiving unfractionated heparin [20].

Regional anaesthesia and intravenous heparin for vascular surgery can be considered under the following conditions:

- After needle or catheter attempt intravenous heparin is delayed by 1 hour.
- Prolonged anticoagulation increases the risk of spinal haematoma, especially in combination with other anticoagulants or thrombolytic agents. If systematic anticoagulation is given when the patient has an epidural catheter, its withdrawn has to be delayed 2-4 hours after discontinuation of heparin, and after the coagulation status is evaluated.
- The catheter is withdrawn one hour before administration of heparin.
- If total daily dose < 10 000 units, there is no contraindication to neuraxial techniques if subcutaneous standard heparin is given. The risk of spinal haematoma with higher doses are uncertain; neurological follow-up is done on an individual basis and is closely evaluated.
- In patients receiving subcutaneous heparin > 5 days serial platelet counts should be performed.

8.5. Low-Molecular-Weight Heparin (LMWH)

Enoxaparin was the first approved LMWH by the FDA in 1993. Between 1993-1997, 30 cases of spinal haematoma were seen in patients receiving LMWH and undergoing spinal or epidural anaesthesia. In 1997, the FDA has started to investigate these cases. In addition, all LMWH and heparinoid manufacturers were warned [9].

Anesthesia and Anticoagulation Neuroaxial consensus conference (1998) described 45 spinal haematoma cases associated with LMWH, in 40 of these patients neuraxial anaesthesia was implicated. Severe radicular back pain was not manifest symptoms, but most patients had incipient numbness, weakness, and bowel or bladder dysfunction. Median time between the treatment start with LMWH and neurological dysfunction development was 3 days, and the mean time between onset of symptoms and laminectomy was more than 24 hours. Bad or good neurological recovery were seen in less than 1/3 patients.

The risk of spinal haematoma due to LMWH, neuraxial techniques, and the prevalence of reported cases, with continuous epidural anaesthesia was reported in approximately 1/3000, with spinal anaesthesia 1:40,000. However, the cases are probably more. About 60 cases have been reported between the years of 1993-1998 by the FDA. The Second Consensus Conference 1998-2002, reported 13 spinal haematoma cases related to neuraxial block. In addition to LMWH, 5 patients received ketorolac, one patient was taking ibuprofen, and one patient received intravenous unfractionated heparin. Spinal anaesthesia in 3 cases, and 10 patients underwent epidural anaesthesia while receiving LMWH. Thus, the reported characteristics of

http://dx.doi.org/10.5772/58702

patients are supported previously recommendations that epidural catheter withdrawal before starting LMWH thromboprophylaxis and other antiplatelet or anticoagulant medication [9]. (Table 4).

Patients factors	Female gender
	Elderly
	Ankylosing spondylitis or spinal stenosis
	Renal failure
Anaesthesia factors	Traumatic needle/catheter placement
	More risk in epidural compared with spinal technique
	Epidural catheter placement during LMWH therapy
LMWH dosage factors	Early preoperative (or intraoperative) LMWH therapy
	Early postoperative LMWH therapy
	Concomitant antiplatelet or anticoagulant medications
	Twice daily LMWH administration

Table 4. Patient, anaesthetic, and LMWH dosing variables associated with spinal haematoma [7]

The effect of renal function cannot be completely evaluated. The anticoagulant effect increased in serious renal failure and half-life is prolonged from 4-6 hours to 16 hours [22].

Efforts to determine the indications for LMWH are continuing. LMWH is not a good choice for patients receiving chronic warfarin therapy, and is indicated for pregnant women, in patients with prosthetic heart valve and atrial fibrillation, and in patients with a history and existing hypercoagulable states. LMWH dose for the treatment of DVT is higher than dosage of prophylaxis. The needle must be inserted at least 24 hours after last dose [9].

8.5.1. Regional anaesthesia management in patients receiving LMWH [20]

Perioperative management of patients receiving LMWH requires coordination and communication. In addition, even if there is a protocol the patient dose may not be closely followed. LMWH is not recommended with other antiplatelet or oral anticoagulant drugs.

Preoperative LMWH

- Neuraxial techniques should be applied at least 10-12 hours after thromboprophylaxis dose and 24 hours after high therapeutic dose of the LMWH.

Postoperative LMWH

- Two doses per day, the first dose of LMWH should be given at least 24 hours after the operation, regardless of the anaesthetic technique, and only if there is adequate hemostasis.

- Remove the catheter before starting LMWH thromboprophylaxis.

- The first dose of LMWH should be given at least 2 hours after withdrawal of catheter, and after 24 hours insertion of needle or catheter.
- The interval between the insertion of needle or catheter with the first dose of LMWH should be 6-8 hours. The other dose should not be given within 24 hours after the first dose.

Antiplatelet medications

Antiplatelet drugs includes the nonsteroidal anti-inflammatory drugs (NSAIDs), thienopyridine, and glycoprotein IIb/IIIa inhibitors, seldom used as agents for primary thromboprophylaxis. It is important to note the pharmacologic differences among the drugs with antiplatelet effects. Many orthopaedic patients are chronic NSAIDs (aspirin, ibuprofen, ketorolac, and naproxen) users. Three of the 61 reported patients who developed spinal haematoma after spinal or epidural anaesthesia were taking antiplatelet therapy. Many studies of these drugs showed that they are relatively safe for neuraxial block in obstetric, surgical, or pain clinic patients [10, 23]. Clinician also should be alert in heparinized patients who also take antiplatelet agents as possible increased risk of spinal haematoma. Ticlopidine and clopidogrel are from thienopyridine group, and are also platelet aggregation inhibitors. These agents inhibit the platelet-fibrinogen binding and then impair platelet-platelet interaction [9]. This effect is irreversible during the platelets life time. Platelet dysfunction lasts 5-7 days for clopidogrel and 10-14 days after ticlopidine. Clopidogrel'in completely normal clotting dose range need not secure due to the block. Prasugrel is a new thienopyridine drug and inhibits platelets faster and sustained. It is used only for percutaneous coronary intervention in acute coronary syndromes in the United States of America.

Platelet glycoprotein IIb/IIIa receptor antagonists (abciximab, eptifibatide and tirofiban) impair platelet aggregation, platelet-fibrinogen binding and platelet-platelet interaction. Time to normal platelet aggregation following discontinuation of therapy ranges from 8 hours (eptifibatide, tirofiban) to 24 to 48 hours (abciximab). During therapy with GP IIb/IIIa antagonists, labeling precautions recommend that puncture of noncompressible sites and "epidural" procedures be avoided [9].

8.5.2. Regional anaesthesia management in patients receiving antiplatelet drugs [20].

- If antiplatelet drugs are taken together with other anticoagulants, bleeding risk is high.
- NSAIDs alone does not a significant risk factor for spinal haematoma in epidural or spinal anaesthesia.
- Platelet function should be return to normal before neuroaxial block in patients receiving ticlopidine, clopidogrel, and platelet GP IIb/IIIa receptor antagonists. Platelet aggregation was returning to normal after discontinuation of the drug: 14 days for ticlopidine; 5-7 days for clopidogrel; 7-10 days for prasugrel. The effects of GP IIb/IIIa inhibitors are terminated between 8 hours (eptifibatide and tirofiban) with 48 hours (abciximab).

http://dx.doi.org/10.5772/58702

8.6. Herbal medications

The use of herbal products in surgical patients is frequent, and sometimes the patients also may disguise their use of them. Polypharmacy and physiological changes lead to morbidity and mortality in the perioperative period. The bleeding may be seen due to garlic, ginkgo, ginseng and ginseng-warfarin interaction. These commercial products are not yet sufficiently under control, therefore, unexpected and adverse reactions may be seen, and in particular, and the anaesthesiologist should be familiar the effects of these agents [9].

Herbal treatment and regional anaesthesia management [20].

- Herbal remedies does not pose any additional risk for spinal haematoma in epidural or spinal anaesthesia. There is not a fully accepted test to assess the adequacy of haemostasis for the herbal products. Inquiry and evaluation should be performed preoperatively. There is no data evaluating the combination of herbal therapy with other anticoagulants. However, an increased risk of bleeding with the drugs that effect on hemostasis system.

8.7. Fondaparinux

Fondaparinux is a synthetic pentasaccharide, the FDA approved in 2001, makes antithrombotic effect by the inhibition of factor Xa. Plasma half-life of 21 hours, 6 hours after the operation is given once daily. Spinal haematomas have not been reported with its use, but it must be used very carefully. The actual risk of spinal haematoma to fondaparinux is unknown.

Fondaparinux and regional anaesthesia management [20].

- Neuraxial techniques should be applied carefully until an adequate clinical information is obtained (single pass through with a needle, the use of atraumatic needle, avoidance from neuraxial catheter). If the precautions are not possible,another method of prevention should be considered.

8.8. Dabigatran

Dabigatran etexilate reversibly inhibits clot bound thrombin. It is a prodrug, gastrointestinal absorption and bioavailability is about 5%. After being absorbed, esterases returned it the active metabolite, dabigatran. A single dose of dabigatran has a half-life of 8 hours, with multiple doses is 17 hours. Daily dose of the drug is suitable. It is contraindicated in patients with renal failure, because 80 % of the drug is excreted unchanged from the kidney. Spinal haematomas are not reported but currently data are insufficient. It is currently used only in non-valvular atrial fibrillation [7].

Management of regional anaesthesia in patients receiving dabigatran [20].

- Dabigatran should be discontinued 7 days before the neuraxial block, because of the long half-life, and irreversible effect. Neuraxial catheters should be withdrawn at least 6 hours prior to initiation of treatment with dabigatran [22].

8.9. Rivaroxaban

Rivaroxaban is a potent, selective and reversible, orally active factor Xa inhibitor. Oral bioavailability is approximately 80%. Maximum inhibitory effect is seen in 1-4 hours and the inhibition lasts 12 hours. Antithrombotic effect is measured by PT, aPTT, and Heptest. It is excreted through kidney and intestine, therefore in patients with renal failure is contraindicated. The half-life is 9 hours, but in the elderly last up to 13 hours. Clinical studies showed that rivaroxaban (5-40 mg a day, the first dose 6-8 hours after surgery) a similar effect with enoxaparin (40 mg given 12 hours before surgery). Although spinal haematoma is not reported, it must be use cautiously because of the longer half-life [10].

Management of regional anaesthesia in patients receiving rivaroxaban [20].

- According to the European guidelines, neuroaxial block can be applied after 22 to 26 hours of discontinuation of rivaroxaban. If there is renal failure this interval will be longer. Neuraxial catheters are contraindicated. Postoperative rivaroxaban treatment should be started at least 4-6 hours after the spinal block [22].

8.10. Peripheral nerve blocks and plexus blocks

It is known that the most important serious complication of neuraxial blocks is spinal haematoma, but the risk is not identified for plexus and peripheral blocks. Few serious complications have been reported. In patients received antiplatelet or anticoagulant agents, major bleeding is reported after lumbar sympathetic block, or psoas compartment block. Neurological damage has not been reported. The Neuroaxial Anesthesia and Anticoagulation Consensus Statement are also used for the peripheral and plexus blocks [9, 10]

9. Diagnosis and treatment

In the differential diagnosis of postoperative new or progressive neurologic symptoms, surgical neuropraxia, prolonged or exaggerated neuraxial block, anterior spinal artery syndrome, epidural abscess, recurrence and existing undiagnosed neurological condition, neurological disorders and spinal haematoma should be considered. Immediate post-operative onset of symptoms is rare. Spinal haematomas rarely can be seen as "prolonged" in the form of blocks [5, 6]. The time between the start of thromboprophylaxis with the entry of the needle is important for neurological dysfunction. Complete paralysis develops within 10-15 hours after the start of neurological deficits. Clinical assessment should be focused on the recognition of reversible or treatable causes. Thus, if any new or progressive neurological symptoms are seen during epidural analgesia, infusion must be promptly stopped (catheter is left) and the local anaesthetic effect and of volume effect is ruled out. If the neurological deficit is due tothelocal anaesthetic and/or volume effects, the deficit is often return quickly,and it should be noted. Neurological recovery is due to early diagnosis and intervention, radiographic imaging, preferably MRI should be done as soon as possible. In terms of the need for emergency surgery, neurosurgery consultation should be requested immediately. Inter-

http://dx.doi.org/10.5772/58702

estingly, all spinal haematomas do not require emergency surgery, spontaneous healing have also been reported [5, 6]. However, the decision of an emergent surgery or observation belongs to the neurosurgeon. Neurological outcome for most patients are worse in all series. In addition, if there is more than 8 hours after onset of the symptoms, a full recovery usually has not been realized. Generally, bleeding after peripheral techniques is less common than neuraxial haematoma, and often appears as hypovolemia not neural deficit. The decide for surgery or observation for neuraxial haematoma or bleeding is based on the presence and severity of neural deficit.

10. Summary and conclusion

Spinal hematoma is a haemorrhage in the spinal or epidural space that develops with forming a heterogeneous group of disorders. Haematoma can be acute, chronic, spontaneous, traumatic or iatrogenic. It is especially related to medication or disease associated with coagulopathy. MRI is a special importance in diagnosis. Delay of surgery may rapidly worsen the clinical outcome, so the surgery should be done urgently.

Spinal haematomas are rare and potentially reversible spinal cord compression. Early diagnosis is essential for a full recovery. Spinal haematomas can occur in the absence of identifiable risk factors. The clinician should be alert for the new neurological signs. Spinal cord and root compression are potentially reversible. If the treatment is done quickly healing is complete. Continuous surveillance of risk identification, assessment and training up to date information for the physician should be done constantly for spinal and epidural blocks. The introduction of new anticoagulants and antiplatelet agents, and the complex balance between thromboembolic events and hemorrhagic complications with regional anaesthesia or analgesia requirement requires an evaluation of the indications for patient. Thus, the antithrombotic therapy in patients receiving spinal or epidural anaesthesia or analgesia, timing of catheter removal should be evaluated basis on the patient's situations. If there is an unacceptable risk, alternative anaesthesia or analgesia techniques should be considered. The patient's coagulation status should be optimized and the level of anticoagulation should be carefully monitored during epidural catheterization. If there is a significant increase in the risk of spinal haematoma, the catheter should not be removed. Identification of risk factors and the publication of the guidelines does not eliminate the complication of spinal haematoma. It is reported that spinal haematoma may develop in patients treated in accordance with the guidelines [24, 25]. United States [10] Europe [26] and the Nordic countries [27, 28] have published guidelines. Closely monitored of the patient to detect early neurological dysfunction is very important to recognize and attempt to fast decompression. Not only try to prevent of spinal haematoma, but also should be focused to make the best of the neurological consequences [7, 10].

Summary of the clinical key points

1. The clinician should have a high index of suspicion at all times in any patient who has undergone spinal anaesthesia and who exhibits any sign or symptom of a neuraxial haematoma

2. Adequate monitoring, follow-up, and immediately treatment are essential in patients on anticoagulants who are receiving neuraxial blocks
3. Early recognition of epidural haematoma
4. Physical examination: vibration and position ability in the lower extremities. Pain, temperature, and light touch (last sensory modalities), Assessing rectal tone.
5. If a new or progressive neurologic deficit are observed during epidural analgesia infusion, it requires immediate discontinuation and the catheter is left in place
6. Urgent radiographic diagnostic studies: MRI (more sensitive and preferred method), Conventional CT, conventional angiography, myelography and CT
7. Differential diagnosis: Epidural abscess, spinal cord disease, neoplasia, muscular or ligamentous injury related to needle placement, postoperative surgical neuropraxia, prolonged or exaggerated neuroaxial block, anterior spinal artery syndrome, and pre-existing undiagnosed neurological disorder
8. Emergency neurosurgical evaluation for surgical decompression.

Author details

R. Hakan Erbay[1], Nimet Senoglu[1] and Habib Atalay[2]

1 Izmir Tepecik Training and Research Hospital, Izmir, Turkey

2 Pamukkale University Medical Faculty, Denizli, Turkey

References

[1] Erbay RH. Epidural / Spinal Hematom Tani ve Tedavisi (Epidural or Spinal Hematoma: Diagnosis and Treatment). Guldogus F, Gurkan Y (Eds). Rejyonal Anestezi. Nobel Tip Kitabevleri (Medical Publishing), Istanbul, Turkey, Chapter 26; 473-84; 2013.

[2] Grejda S, Ellis K, Arino P. Paraplegia following spinal anesthesia in a patient with chronic renal failure. Reg Anesth 1989;14:155–157.

[3] Shah R, Kaye AD, Kaye A, Tsai JY. Anticoagulation and Regional Anesthesia. In: Kaye AD, Urman RD, Vadivelu N (Eds): Essentials of Regional Anesthesia. Springer, New York, 158-168, 2012.

[4] Jabri RS, Deschner S, Benzon HT. Part XI. Neurologic Complications of Regional Anesthesia: Chapter 71. Diagnosis & Management of Intraspinal, Epidural, & Peripheral

http://dx.doi.org/10.5772/58702

Nerve Hematoma. In: Hadzic A. (Ed) Textbook of Regional Anesthesia and Acute Pain Management. McGraw-Hill Companies. Printed in China. 2007.

[5] Vandermeulen EP, Van Aken H, Vermylen J. Anticoagulants and spinal–epidural anesthesia. Anesth Analg 1994; 79: 1165–77.

[6] Moen V, Dahlgren N, Irestedt L. Severe neurological complications after central neuraxial blockades in Sweden 1990–1999. Anesthesiology 2004; 101: 950–9.

[7] Horlocker TT. Regional anaesthesia in the patient receiving antithrombotic and antiplatelet therapy. Br J Anaesth. 2011;107 (S1): 96-106.

[8] Li SL, Wang DX, Ma D. Epidural hematoma after neuraxial blockade: a retrospective report from China. Anesth Analg 2010;111:1322-4.

[9] Horlocker TT, Wedel DJ, Benzon H, et al. Regional anesthesia in the anticoagulated patient: defining the risks (the second ASRA Consensus Conference on Neuroaxial Anesthesia and Anticoagulation). Reg Anesth Pain Med 2003; 28: 172–97.

[10] Horlocker TT, Wedel DJ, Rowlingson JC, et al. Regional anesthesia in the patient receiving antithrombotic or thrombolytic therapy: American Society of Regional Anesthesia and Pain Medicine Evidence-Based Guidelines (Third Edition). Reg Anesth Pain Med 2010; 35: 64–10.

[11] Sinatra RS, Froicu DB: Chapter 12. Regional Anesthesia Complications. In: Ruskin KJ, Rosenbaum SH (eds): Anesthesia Emergencies. Oxford University Press, New York, 298-313, 2011.

[12] Pahapill PA, Lownie SP: Conservative treatment of acute spontaneous spinal epidural hematoma. Can J Anaesth 1998;25:159–163.

[13] Taniguchi LU, Pahl FH, Lúcio JE, et al. Complete motor recovery after acute paraparesis caused by spontaneous spinal epidural hematoma: case report. BMC Emerg Med 2011, 27;11:10.

[14] Wulf H. Epidural anaesthesia and spinal haematoma. Can J Anaesth.1996;43(12): 1260-71.

[15] Lawton M, Porter R, Heiserman J, et al: Surgical management of spinal epidural hematoma: Relationship between surgical timing and neurological outcome. J Neurosurg 1995;83:1–7.

[16] Hejazi N, Thaper PY, Hassler W: Nine cases of nontraumatic spinal epidural hematoma. Neurol Med Chir 1998;38:718–23.

[17] Ho AM, Chung DC, Joynt GM. Neuraxial blockade and hematoma in cardiac surgery: estimating the risk of a rare adverse event that has not (yet) occurred. Chest. 2000;117(2):551–5.

[18] Raj PP, Shah RV, Kaye AD, Denaro S, Hoover JM. Bleeding risk in interventional pain practice: assessment, management, and review of the literature. Pain Physician. 2004;7(1):3–51.

[19] Geerts WH, Bergqvist D, Pineo GF, et al. Prevention of venous thromboembolism: American College of Chest Physicians Evidence-Based Clinical Practice Guidelines (8th Edition). Chest 2008; 133: 381S–453S.

[20] Horlocker TT, Birnbach DJ, Connis RT, et al. Practice advisory for the prevention, diagnosis, management of infectious complications associated with neuraxial techniques: a report by the American Society of Anesthesiologists Task Force on infectious complications associated with neuraxial techniques. Anesthesiology 2010; 112: 530–45.

[21] Liu SS, Buvanendran A, Viscusi ER, et al. Uncomplicated removal of epidural catheters in 4365 patients with international normalized ratio greater than 1.4 during initiation of warfarin therapy. Reg Anesth Pain Med 2011; 36: 231–5.

[22] Gogarten W, Vandermeulen E, Van Aken H, Kozek S, Llau JV, Samama CM. Regional anaesthesia and antithrombotic agents: recommendations of the European Society of Anaesthesiology Eur J Anaesthesiol 2010; 27: 999–1015.

[23] Horlocker TT, Bajwa ZH, Ashraf Z, et al. Risk assessment of hemorrhagic complications associated with nonsteroidal antiinflammatory medications in ambulatory pain clinic patients undergoing epidural steroid injection. Anesth Analg 2002; 95: 1691–7.

[24] Elwood D, Koo C. PM R. 2009 Apr;1(4):389-96. Intraspinal Hematoma Following Neuraxial Anesthesia and Low-Molecular-Weight Heparin in Two Patients: Risks and Benefits of Anticoagulation. PM R. 2009 Apr;1(4):389-96.

[25] Gogarten W, Vandermeulen E, Van Aken H, et al. Regional anaesthesia and antithrombotic agents: recommendations of the European Society of Anaesthesiology. Eur J Anaesthesiol. 2010;27(12):999-1015.

[26] Breivik H, Bang U, Jalonen J, Vigfusson G, Alahuhta S, Lagerkranser M. Nordic guidelines for neuraxial blocks in disturbed haemostasis from the Scandinavian Society of Anaesthesiology and Intensive Care Medicine. Acta Anaesthesiol Scand. 2010;54:16-41.

[27] Moen V. Scandinavian guidelines for neuraxial block and disturbed haemostasis: replacing wishful thinking with evidence based caution. Acta Anaesthesiol Scand. 2010;54:6-8.